A WOMAN
DOCTOR'S
GUIDE TO
INFERTILITY

A WOMAN DOCTOR'S GUIDE TO INFERTILITY

Essential Facts and Up-to-the-Minute
Information on the Techniques and
Treatments to Achieve Pregnancy

By

Susan Treiser, M.D., Ph.D.

with

Robin K. Levinson

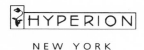

NEW YORK

LIBRARY OF CONGRESS CATALOGING-IN-PUBLICATION DATA

Treiser, Susan.
     A woman doctor's guide to infertility : essential facts and up-to-the-minute information on the techniques and treatments to achieve pregnancy / by Susan Treiser, with Robin K. Levinson. — 1st ed.
          p.   cm.
     Includes bibliographical references and index.
     ISBN 0-7868-8010-4
     1. Infertility—Popular works.   I. Levinson, Robin K.   II. Title.
RC889.T734   1994
616.6'92—dc20   93-31568
                                                                      CIP

FIRST EDITION

10 9 8 7 6 5 4 3 2 1

I dedicate this book to my mother, whose continuous pride in my accomplishments pushed me to limits I did not think possible and who sadly did not live to see the final outcome; to my father, for his quiet but ever present love and support; to my husband, Murray, and children, Mathew and Adam, for allowing me to be "me."

—Susan Treiser

To my husband, Larry, who taught me how to stay hopeful through the darkest days; to my long-awaited daughter, Zoë Mae, who has enriched our lives beyond anything we ever imagined; to my mother and father, Arlene and Alan Lichtenstein, who never pressured me to be anything more than I am; and to Zoë Mae's godmother, Sharon Schlegel, for brimming with love and empathy whenever I needed it most.

—Robin Levinson

CONTENTS

LIST OF ILLUSTRATIONS

INTRODUCTION

Thirty years ago, most people with impaired fertility had few options but to adopt a child or resign themselves to childlessness. Fertility drugs were available, but that fact was not widely known. Like cancer, infertility was talked about in whispered tones, if at all.

Today, infertility treatment innovations make frequent headlines, and the topic is addressed openly among family and friends and on television talk shows. Many books and articles have been written about infertility, and a nationwide support group lobbies state legislatures to mandate insurance coverage for infertility treatment. It's no secret that couples facing infertility in the '90s have a virtual arsenal of weapons to combat this potentially devastating condition.

This book will acquaint you with that arsenal and, we hope, put you on the road to parenthood. You will learn about the delicate, intricate symphony of hormonal events that must play out to foster and support a pregnancy. You will be introduced to the jargon, acronyms, diagnostic tools, surgeries, drugs, and procedures doctors use to help patients overcome infertility. You will get some tips on choosing a physician and coping emotionally, socially, and financially. And you will learn that you have up to a 70 percent chance of becoming pregnant after at least one year of treatment, depending on the complexity of your problem and who your doctor is.

PART I
DISCOVERING
IF YOU'RE
INFERTILE

CHAPTER 1

DEFINING INFERTILITY: MYTHS AND FACTS

If you're like most women, having children is for you a fundamental desire. As a little girl playing with dolls, you fantasized about the day in the distant future when you would become a real mommy. You grew up in a culture that covets children, where cooing adults flock around newborns as predictably as candles flicker on a birthday cake, where graduation ceremonies and weddings were as much a source of pride for your parents as they were for you and your contemporaries.

As you got older, your co-workers, friends, and siblings began having children. You and your husband may have been using birth control for years with the idea of starting a family as soon as your careers were set and there was a nest egg in the bank. You may even have opened a college fund account for your future progeny. If you married relatively late, if you hear the ticking of your so-called "biological time clock," getting pregnant takes on a more urgent demeanor.

The fact that you're reading this book suggests your dream of having a baby is degenerating into a nightmare. The once-mundane act of getting your period may now trigger tears, frustration, depression, and even rage—rage that your body is not doing as you command. You may be questioning your womanhood or your husband's manhood. You may even wonder if God is punishing you for some past sin.

If you've been trying unsuccessfully to become pregnant for a year or more, you may have some form of infertility. And you are far from alone. Infertility, defined as the inability to conceive a child naturally, affected an estimated 4.9 million individuals—almost 2.5 million couples—in this country in 1988, according to the most recent data available from the National Center for Health Statistics. Viewed another way, about 15 percent of people in their childbearing years, ages 15 to 44, or about 1 in 12 Americans, cannot bear a child because of problems with their own reproductive system, their spouse's, or a combination of both.

There are two basic kinds of infertility—primary and secondary—although the diagnostic approach and available treatments for both are the same. If you've never been pregnant and have not conceived after 12 months of having regular, unprotected intercourse, you may be one of the estimated 2.2 million women and men experiencing primary infertility. If you've been pregnant before but are unable to become or stay pregnant again, your general diagnosis is secondary infertility, a condition affecting about 2.7 million women and men.

According to the Center for Health Statistics study, the number of women with primary infertility doubled between 1965 and 1982. The scope of the problem remained relatively fixed between 1982 and 1988.

During that same time frame, the number of people seeking infertility treatment snowballed. The number of infertility specialists has also risen dramatically over the years. Membership in the American Fertility Society, one of several professional organizations representing reproduction specialists, has ballooned from 100 members at its inception in 1944 to more than 11,000 physicians and scientists from 50 states and more than 118 foreign countries today. The society calls itself the "fastest growing subspecialty group in the medical field."

Some 1 million Americans and their insurers spend more than $1 billion a year on infertility treatments, according to government estimates. The number of people seeking a professional consultation for infertility doubled between 1981 and 1982 alone, according to researcher William D. Mosher, Ph.D., of the Center for Health Statistics Division of Vital Statistics. In 1987, there were fewer than 50 in-vitro fertilization (IVF) clinics in the United States. Today, there are more than 200.

Doctors sometimes use another term to describe difficulty getting and staying pregnant—"impaired fecundity." Infertility and impaired fecundity are not to be confused with "sterility," which means you cannot conceive under any circumstances.

Unless you already know you are sterile owing to bilateral oophorectomy (surgical removal of both ovaries), or chemotherapy or radiation therapy, you probably don't know you have a fertility problem until you begin trying to get pregnant. Most doctors won't begin diagnostic testing until you have deliberately tried to get pregnant for at least six months if you are over 35 and at least a year if you are younger. Doctors usually suspect a fertility problem if you suffered three or more first-trimester miscarriages.

Also take into account your health, since certain infections can hamper your ability to have children. Ask your doctor or pharmacist whether a prescription drug your husband or you are taking can affect reproduction. Illnesses such as alcoholism or even the flu can lower your husband's sperm count for as long as three months after recovery. You both should refrain from using recreational drugs such as marijuana and cocaine while you are trying to conceive—and, of course, after you do.

Try to achieve a normal body weight before attempting to have a baby. Obesity or insufficient body fat can make you ovulate irregularly or not at all.

How your body fat is distributed also can have an impact on your fertility. A recent study of 500 healthy female patients in a Netherlands fertility clinic suggested that apple-shaped women

—those with waists bigger than their hips—were only half as likely to get pregnant as were pear-shaped women. The study, published in the February 20, 1993, issue of the *British Medical Journal,* looked at healthy, primarily normal-weight women ages 20 to 42 who were being artificially inseminated with donor sperm. "Body-fat distribution in women of reproductive age seems to have more impact on fertility than age or obesity," the researchers concluded. The reasons for their findings were unclear, however.

WHY SO MANY PEOPLE
SEEK TREATMENT

The steady growth of the infertility industry can be attributed in large part to demographics. For starters, the baby-boom generation (those born between 1946 and 1964) is well into the childbearing years. According to U.S. census data, the median age of a first-time bride was 20½ in 1970 and almost 24 in 1988. The number of never-married women between ages 25 and 29 more than tripled between 1970 and 1991, from 10.5 percent to 32.3 percent. In the 30 to 34 age bracket, the number of never-married women more than tripled, from 6.2 percent in 1970 to 18.7 percent in 1991.

Even after marriage, more and more women are delaying pregnancy in order to pursue higher education and careers. Women who prefer to be full-time homemakers often are forced into the workplace to help make ends meet. Between 1974 and 1978, only 4.5 percent of babies were born to mothers older than 35. In the late '80s and early '90s, that percentage had risen to about 6.5 percent. By 2000, about 10 percent of all births are projected to be by women older than 35.

While few of us would trade the grounds and options we have gained as a result of the modern women's movement, most are shocked to discover that delaying pregnancy may result in a fertility problem. The average woman's fertility potential gradually decreases after age 35, although women can have a perfectly healthy baby at age 40 or older. According to a 1988 study by Mosher and colleagues, the percentage of childless couples with impaired fecundity increased from 8 percent in the 15- to 24-year-old age group to 36 percent in couples between ages 35 and 44. In fact, the chance of conceiving naturally in your mid-40s is only about 5 percent, while the miscarriage rate is almost 50 percent. Aside from the problem of aging eggs (we're born with all the eggs we'll ever produce), there are the risks associated with multiple sex partners. People who spend more of their adult lives single tend to have more than one lover. The subsequent rise in sexually transmitted diseases has left many of these women with pelvic inflammatory disease (PID). Even if properly treated, PID may leave a legacy of scar tissue in and around reproductive organs, which can impair fertility. Because PID may have no symptoms, many women never even know they had it.

Women whose mothers took the anti-miscarriage drug, diethylstilbestrol (DES) in the 1950s and '60s are in or approaching the latter stage of their childbearing years. DES was banned when it was discovered that it caused reproductive problems in many children exposed to the drug in the womb. While a DES-caused abnormality won't necessarily prevent conception, it can make it difficult for a fertilized egg to implant and grow. This raises the incidence of miscarriage.

Some researchers believe that pollution and the preponderance of chemicals and toxins in our environment may be responsible for depressing sperm counts. It was reported in late 1992 that women who make semiconductor chips for a living may have a higher risk of miscarriage, because of the solvents used in the manufacturing process. Cigarette smoking also has been linked to fertility problems in women.

According to the American Fertility Society, many doctors believe that women who have never been pregnant are more likely to have a fertility-threatening disease called endometriosis. Normally, tissue known as endometrium builds up on the inside of the uterus each month to prepare for a potential pregnancy. In endometriosis, pieces of endometrium also implant themselves outside the uterus. These implants can themselves block an egg from reaching the sperm or trigger the formation of scar tissue in the pelvic cavity.

THE ETHICS OF TREATMENT

When pregnancy doesn't come as easily as couples expect, as many as 75 percent will seek medical care. Some are lured by the potential of reproductive miracles they have heard about in the mass media.

The first explosion of news reports came with the birth of the world's first "test-tube baby," Louise Brown of Britain, in 1978. Publicity bloomed again when the first American test-tube baby, Elizabeth Jordan Carr, was born on December 28, 1981, in Norfolk, Virginia. Then there was the sustained coverage in the mid-1980s of Mary Beth Whitehead, the surrogate mother who fought to maintain custody of the infant "Baby M," whom she gave birth to under contract with another couple.

In November 1992, a 62-year-old Sicilian widow announced she became pregnant through artificial insemination with sperm that had been collected from her husband and frozen before he died. That case came on the heels of twin girls born to Mary Shearing, a 53-year-old California grandmother. Shearing's babies were conceived in a petri dish with sperm from her husband and eggs donated by a 20-year-old and transferred into Shearing's womb. As of early 1993, at least two grandmothers had given birth to their own grandchildren conceived in a laboratory with eggs provided by their daughters.

Even entertainment television is talking about infertility. An "L.A. Law" episode, based on a real case in Tennessee, depicted a divorced man who won an injunction to prevent frozen embryos, conceived with his sperm, from being implanted into his ex-wife's uterus. According to Professor John A. Robertson, J.D., of the University of Texas School of Law, these types of lawsuits can probably be avoided if both partners sign an agreement at the time their embryos are frozen. The agreement should spell out what they would like to happen to the embryos in case of divorce, separation, or death. "It is reasonable to assume that such agreements would be legally binding," Robertson wrote in the April 1991 issue of the medical journal *Fertility and Sterility*.

As reproductive technology advances, the web of ethical and moral dilemmas grows more intricate. In an interview aired on National Public Radio's "Talk of the Nation" in December 1992, Arthur Caplan, then director of the Center for Biomedical Ethics at the University of Minnesota, raised the issue of a child's right to know that he or she was conceived as a result of donor eggs, donor embryos, or donor sperm. Indeed, at least one group of adult children conceived through donor insemination has already formed in the United States to help members track down their biological fathers, a difficult if not impossible task since the vast majority of sperm donors are guaranteed anonymity by sperm banks. Aside from satisfying their curiosity, Caplan said, children conceived through donor insemination may be seeking a complete genetic history—information that is becoming increasingly pertinent as researchers learn more and more about links between heredity and disease. The situation could even become a life-or-death matter should the child ever need a bone-marrow transplant. Caplan foresees a time when children conceived through donor technology may band together, as adoptive children have, to lobby for their rights.

Of more immediate concern, the Roman Catholic Church in a 1992 catechism labeled artificial insemination and other non-natural means of conception a sin. This declaration is a potential source of stress for infertile Roman Catholics, who must reconcile their religious beliefs with their desire to have children before deciding whether to pursue treatment.

The potential of abuse and incompetence by infertility clinics is another source of worry. In a 1990 report titled "Quality Assurance in Reproductive Technologies," the Ethics Committee of the American Fertility Society points out that patients may be unable to adequately judge the quality of an in-vitro fertilization program. "It would be possible for a clinic to have no successes without the patients ever realizing it," the committee wrote. "For example, with respect to IVF, the current maximum pregnancy rate is below 30 percent per treatment cycle. Couples who failed to achieve pregnancy might believe that they were among the unlucky 70 percent and might not recognize that they had not received adequate care."

The issue of patient vulnerability has been the subject of several newspaper and magazine stories in recent years. These articles point out that because the infertility industry is largely unregulated, some clinics tend to exaggerate their success rates or overtreat patients. That is the exception, however, not the rule.

A March 15, 1992, *New York Times Magazine* article titled "Tales from the Baby Factory" implied that fertility specialists are getting rich from desperate couples who are willing to undergo great physical and financial hardships for a relatively slim shot at becoming pregnant. The article opened with one couple who underwent 20 cycles of treatment with the powerful ovulation drug Pergonal, in conjunction with 13 artificial inseminations, 6 IVF procedures using both the husband's and donor sperm, frozen embryos, and "partial zona drilling," where a minute hole is drilled into the egg's shell to allow a sperm to swim in. For their efforts, the couple got no baby and their bills exceeded $50,000.

That couple's case was extreme, and the article failed to balance their story with anecdotes of people who have been helped through advanced reproductive technologies. The article gave the impression that physicians are enticing these patients with a potential baby. In reality, it is always the couple's decision, not the doctor's, whether to continue treatment. Indeed, most infertility specialists try to dissuade a couple from continuing a treatment that doesn't seem to be working. If a couple hasn't succeeded after three or four in-vitro fertilization procedures, for example, most doctors will encourage them to quit or try a different tack, such as using donor eggs.

The *New York Times* article and others debunking the industry also downplay the fact that, statistically, only 5 percent to 15 percent of couples who enter treatment will wind up resorting to IVF or other advanced assisted reproductive technologies (ART). The rest will become pregnant through less drastic means, or they will abandon treatment because they lack the stamina or the emotional or financial resources to continue. A handful will get pregnant on their own.

In response to consumer complaints about the lack of information on ART programs' pregnancy rates and questions raised by lay people as well as medical specialists on whether fertility patients were being exploited, the federal government has begun to regulate the industry. On October 24, 1992, then President Bush signed into law the Fertility Clinic Success Rate and Certification Act. The act directs the U.S. Department of Health and Human Services to develop a model program for the certification of embryo laboratories, which are used for IVF procedures.

According to a February 1993 article in *Fertility and Sterility,* the law also requires ART programs to provide pregnancy rates to the HHS for yearly publication and distribution to the public upon request beginning in 1995. For the last several years, however, IVF clinic-specific pregnancy rates as well as national pregnancy rates have been compiled and published annually by the American Fertility Society and the Society for Assisted Reproductive Technology.

The article further notes that the College of American Pathologists and the American Fertility Society have jointly developed an accreditation program for embryo labs. That program was launched in mid-1993, while the federal government has until October 24, 1994, to launch its certification program. Infertility patients should be aware that states' participation in the federal lab certification program is voluntary, and "it appears unlikely at this time that many states will decide to implement it in these times of fiscal constraint."

However, the article continues, the legislative process improved the chances for insurance reimbursement for ART procedures and may ultimately help restore federal funding for IVF research, funding that was yanked during the Bush years. "A new day may be dawning in reproductive medicine and biology," wrote the article's authors, Lynne D. Lawrence, of the American Fertility Society, and Zev Rosenwaks, M.D., of Cornell Medical Center.

On the issue of money, the $1 billion spent in 1987 on infertility treatment represented about 0.1 percent of total U.S. health-care expenditures, according to the U.S. Office of Technology Assessment. The emotional toll, meanwhile, is incalculable. Infertility hits people in their peak earning years. Their depression, isolation, humiliation, embarrassment, and other emotional problems can make them less productive at work and in their personal lives. Many couples willingly endure the demands of medical intervention because they are simply unwilling to accept the idea of not having children. With the overall odds approaching 70 percent that medical intervention will help them, they feel their efforts justify the risks. Just ask any previously infertile couple who had a baby after years of costly treatments. Undoubtedly, they'll tell you it was well worth it.

BECOMING INFERTILITY SAVVY

Like any medical problem, infertility is a battle best waged by an informed patient. Accurate information can help you avoid the "bad apple" health-care providers who lie about their success rates or who don't follow scientifically backed protocols. Furthermore, understanding some of the science behind the treatments can help you follow your doctor's instructions and become more involved in your treatment. Knowing which treatments are available to you, what the risks are, whether they hurt, and how much they cost will help you cope emotionally and financially.

Myths Debunked

To prepare yourself for the facts, it's important to put to bed common myths about infertility.

MYTH: If I had an abortion, I can never have a baby.

FACT: If an uncomplicated abortion was done in a safe manner by an experienced licensed practitioner during the first trimester, you can probably conceive and carry a wanted pregnancy to term. However, if there were complications, repeated abortions, or abortions after the first trimester, scar tissue may have formed in your uterus and is impairing fertility.

MYTH: Being stressed out about becoming pregnant prevents conception. Relax, take a vacation, and you'll conceive.

FACT: For most couples, being stressed out is a result of infertility, not a cause, according to Resolve, Inc., a Massachusetts-based information, advocacy, and support network for infertile couples. Fertile couples conceive regardless of their stress level. Even rape victims occasionally become pregnant as a result of their assault. Relaxation can't open blocked fallopian tubes or increase sperm count. Learning to relax has important benefits, though, such as reducing psychological stress to help you endure the rigors of infertility diagnosis and treatment. Swimming, low-impact aerobics, bicycling, meditation, yoga, and the martial arts are great stress-reducers and can help keep your body fit and ready for pregnancy if it occurs.

MYTH: Women with secondary infertility should be satisfied with the child they have and not push their luck.

FACT: Having one child does not necessarily diminish the desire to have another. Indeed, many only children ask for a little brother or sister, and these parents may feel just as desperate as primary infertility patients feel about having a first child. Regardless of what people may tell you, your quest for more children is legitimate.

MYTH: Thirty-five is too old to begin parenting.

FACT: Generally, older couples are more emotionally mature, financially secure, and tend to have more stable marriages. While the risks of infertility, birth defects, and miscarriage do rise after age 35, the odds of conceiving and carrying a healthy baby to term are still in your favor. Prenatal tests, such as amniocentesis, allow older mothers to detect problems early on and raise their chances of having a healthy baby through good prenatal care and proper nutrition. Thanks to hormonal therapy, assisted reproductive technologies, and donor eggs and embryos, even post-menopausal women can carry a baby to term.

MYTH: Women who took birth-control pills have trouble getting pregnant when they go off the pill.

FACT: On the contrary, oral contraceptives, which temporarily halt ovulation, help preserve a woman's store of eggs. It may be prudent, however, to stop taking the pill and use condoms or another form of birth control for six months to allow your natural hormonal output and menstrual cycle to resume before attempting to get pregnant.

MYTH: Using fertility drugs, frozen sperm, or frozen embryos to conceive creates a higher-than-average risk of birth defects.

FACT: No scientific evidence backs this assertion. Babies born after infertility treatment are no more likely to have problems than a baby conceived naturally.

MYTH: If you want a child so badly, you can always adopt. I know a couple who got pregnant after they adopted.

FACT: First of all, adoption is almost always easier in theory than in practice. Waiting lists for a healthy infant, particularly a healthy Caucasian infant, can be one to 10 years or longer through adoption agencies. Adoption can be extremely expensive—$10,000 to $25,000—unless you are willing to adopt an older physically, mentally, or emotionally handicapped child. Even though infertility treatment costs can run that high, well-insured couples find they are paying just a fraction of that amount out-of-pocket. No health insurer covers adoption expenses. Some adoption agencies won't accept couples over age 35 or 40 or couples who have been married less than three years. Also, studies have shown that the pregnancy rate after adoption is about 5 percent—no different from the spontaneous pregnancy rate among previously infertile couples who did not adopt.

CHAPTER 2

CAUSES OF INFERTILITY

Reproduction is an extremely complex enterprise. Your endocrine system must be functioning normally, pumping out the precise levels of hormones at the precise times on a cyclical basis. Your ovaries must be capable of growing at least one egg follicle each month and releasing the egg at the proper juncture in your menstrual cycle. The egg must contain the right amount of genetic material so it can be fertilized and grow into a healthy baby. Your fallopian tubes must be free of obstructions and able to catch and propel the egg toward the uterine cavity.

Your partner's semen must contain many healthy, strong-swimming sperm, and the semen itself must be able to transform from a jelly-like substance to a liquid 30 to 40 minutes after ejaculation. The sperm must be introduced into your reproductive tract during a window of time that may be as brief as 24 hours every 28 or 30 days. Your cervix must be producing enough mucus to protect, nourish, and transport sperm toward the uterus and tubes. Your uterus must be unobstructed and its lining thick and healthy enough to allow a fertilized egg to implant. After conception and implantation, your hormonal system must continue to work smoothly so a placenta can develop and nourish the fetus.

Even a minor, transient glitch can thwart conception. It is easy to see, then, why a fertile couple has only a 20 percent chance of conceiving per cycle, and more than 30 percent of pregnancies are lost spontaneously, usually before the woman realizes she is pregnant. With regular intercourse, however, about 80 percent of fertile couples will conceive within 12 months.

Infertility can stem from a myriad of causes. For about 40 percent of couples, the fertility problem lies within the woman; for another 40 percent, a male factor is the source. For as many as 20 percent of couples, the problem lies within both partners. In some cases, one or both partners are experiencing multiple problems.

Obviously, the number and severity of your problems help determine whether you and your partner will be able to have a baby. Even a single, severe problem can make achieving pregnancy difficult.

Infertility can stem from anatomical, physiological, or hormonal abnormalities. Certain bacterial infections, toxic exposures, alcohol, and drugs (prescription and illicit), as well as chemotherapy and radiation, have been found to diminish fertility, as can certain diseases. Despite the many known sources of infertility, doctors are unable to diagnose the cause in about 15 percent of couples. These couples' diagnosis is "unexplained infertility."

THE REPRODUCTIVE ENDOCRINE SYSTEM

The endocrine system describes the secretion and interplay of hormones throughout the body and the glands responsible for producing the hormones. Hormones are the chemicals that regulate most internal functions, including digestion, temperature, sexual development, and, of course, reproduction. Hormones are secreted into the bloodstream and carried to their target areas. Some hormones serve only to stimulate certain glands to produce other hormones.

The two primary female hormones are estrogen and progesterone, both of which are secreted by the ovaries. At puberty, estrogen levels increase to spur the growth of secondary sex characteristics, such as breasts and widening hips. Estrogen also stimulates the hypothalamus, a gland situated at the base of the brain, to produce gonadotropin-releasing hormone (GnRH), which is normally secreted in a pulsating fashion. GnRH, in turn, tells the nearby pituitary gland to secrete follicle-stimulating hormone (FSH) and luteinizing hormone (LH), which stimulate the ovary to produce a fluid-filled sac, or follicle, containing an egg. The mature follicle produces more estrogen, which then acts to turn off the stimulation of further egg production by inhibiting GnRH, FSH, and LH secretion.

About midway through the menstrual cycle, when the egg has ripened and is ready to be expelled into the fallopian tube, the hypothalamus tells the pituitary to produce a surge of LH, which spurs the follicle to release the egg. Finger-like appendages at the top of the fallopian tubes capture the egg, and millions of tiny hair-like structures called cilia beat rapidly to propel the egg toward the uterus. Meanwhile, the empty follicle, known as the corpus luteum, pumps out both estrogen and progesterone. Under progesterone's influence, the endometrium, or uterine lining, grows thick as it prepares to receive the egg. If the egg is fertilized, the corpus luteum continues to produce progesterone, which helps the endometrium support the pregnancy. If the egg is not fertilized, the corpus luteum deteriorates after about 12 days, and the endometrium is flushed from the body during the woman's period. Named for the hormones that dominate at the time, the first half of the menstrual cycle is known as the "follicular phase," and the second half is called the "luteal phase."

Unlike women, who are born with a finite number of about 400,000 eggs, men are constantly producing new sperm, which have their own life cycle. As in women, the reproductive system in men is orchestrated by the pituitary. The pituitary secretes hormones that instruct the testicles to produce sperm and the male hormone testosterone. At puberty, testosterone stimulates beard growth, a lowering of the voice, and other secondary sex characteristics. The man's pituitary also secretes FSH and LH, but not in cycles, as it does in women.

Immature sperm cells arise in tiny, tube-like structures, called seminiferous tubules, in the testicles. As they mature, these round cells begin to develop a distinct head and tail, somewhat like a tadpole. The tail is the engine, designed to move the sperm through the female reproductive tract. In a healthy sperm cell, the head contains all the genes needed to fertilize an egg. The maturation process takes about 72 days.

As they mature, the sperm leave the testicle through a narrow, 12- to 18-foot coiled tube called the epididymis. The seminal vesicles, the prostate gland, as well as Cowper's glands (located at the base of the penis), all contribute fluids that make up semen. Both the semen and the mature sperm empty first into a tube called the vas deferens and then into the urethra, which carries the mixture out through the penis during ejaculation. Even though more than 150 million sperm (ideally) are expelled during a single ejaculation, the sperm comprise only a small percentage of the total semen volume.

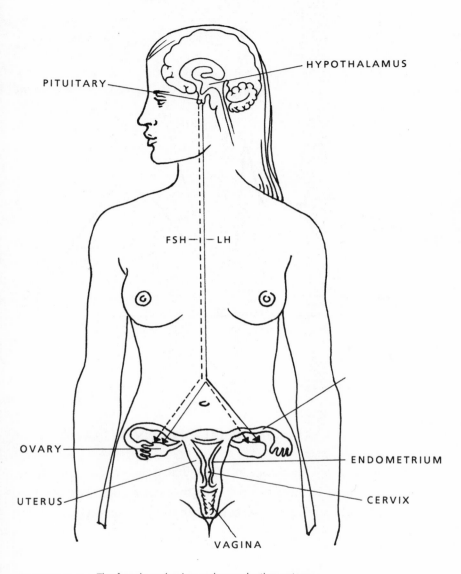

FIGURE 1 The female endocrine and reproductive systems.

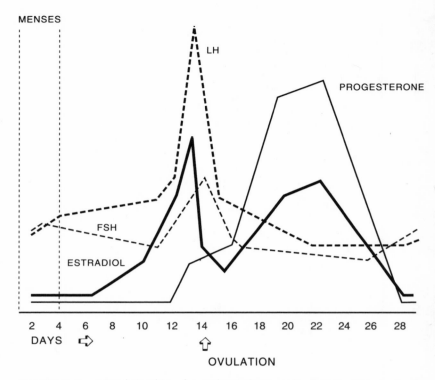

FIGURE 2   Interrelationships of reproductive hormone levels during the menstrual cycle.

WHAT CAN GO WRONG IN WOMEN?

The uterus. The fallopian tubes. The ovaries. The endocrine system. All are subject to problems that can make getting pregnant difficult or impossible, even with medical or surgical intervention.

ENDOMETRIOSIS

One of the most common causes of female infertility is endometriosis, which afflicts about 7 percent of the overall female population but has been reported in 25 percent to 50 percent of infertile women. Symptoms range from severe cramping during

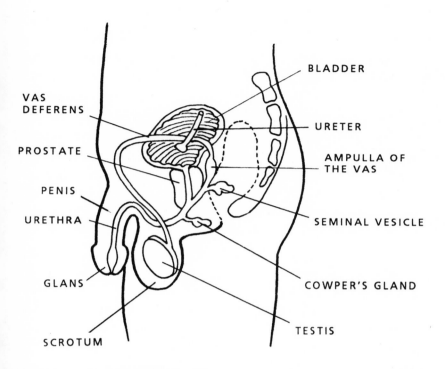

VAS
DEFERENS

PROSTATE

PENIS

URETHRA

GLANS

SCROTUM

BLADDER

URETER

AMPULLA OF
THE VAS

SEMINAL VESICLE

COWPER'S GLAND

TESTIS

FIGURE 3   Male reproductive anatomy.

menstruation to pain during intercourse, or there may be no
pain at all. The disease causes pieces of the endometrium, or
uterine lining, to migrate or grow outside the uterus, implanting
themselves on ovaries, fallopian tubes, or elsewhere in the pelvic
cavity. In rare instances, the endometrium grows in distant
places, such as the lungs.

   The cause or causes of endometriosis are not fully understood, although the condition tends to run in families. One
probable cause is "retrograde menstruation," where some of the
uterine lining flows into the fallopian tubes and spills into the
pelvic region. What triggers retrograde menstruation is a mys-
tery.

Like normal endometrium, the displaced endometrial tissue grows each month under the influence of estrogen and progesterone. Since it has nowhere to go while the normal endometrium flows out of the body, the bleeding of displaced endometrium can irritate reproductive organs and ultimately bind them in scar tissue. Scar tissue, or adhesions, may interfere with reproduction by, for example, pulling a fallopian tube away from the ovary, or blocking or binding the tube. The risk of infertility and the effectiveness of treatment both may depend on where the endometriosis is and its severity. Some people have minimal amounts of endometriosis without any evidence of scar tissue yet have difficulty conceiving.

HORMONAL IMBALANCE

Hormonal imbalances affect up to one-quarter of infertile women. If the pituitary produces insufficient follicle-stimulating hormone, the woman will not produce an egg follicle. If there is no surge of luteinizing hormone, the egg will not be released. If these imbalances happen sporadically, the condition is called "ovulatory dysfunction." Ovulatory dysfunction is far more common than "anovulation," a condition where a woman never ovulates. Even if ovulation is occurring, insufficient progesterone from the corpus luteum will render the endometrium incapable of supporting a fertilized egg. When this happens, the woman has what's known as a "luteal phase defect."

Reasons for hormonal imbalances are not always clear. In a minority of cases, there is a tiny, benign tumor in the pituitary gland hindering its function. Thyroid disease, anorexia nervosa, stress, and polycystic ovarian disease are other possible culprits. As you will see in Chapter 5, hormonal therapy is quite effective in correcting hormonal imbalances for the vast majority of women.

Professional dancers and other extremely athletic women

tend to ovulate irregularly or not at all, probably because of their lack of adequate body fat. If you are involved in heavy exercise, curtail your activity while you are trying to get pregnant.

PELVIC INFLAMMATORY DISEASE

About $3 billion a year is spent treating pelvic inflammatory disease (PID) in the United States. Its primary cause: sexually transmitted diseases. There are about 12 million new cases of sexually transmitted disease and 1 million cases of PID reported each year to the Federal Centers for Disease Control. About 12.5 percent of these infections lead to scar tissue in the fallopian tubes. Tubal scarring can cause blockages that may result in ectopic pregnancy (pregnancy outside the womb). Women who smoke are believed to be especially vulnerable to scarring from PID because smoking slows down the healing process (see "Smoking" entry later in this chapter).

The most common sexually transmitted organisms are gonorrhea, chlamydia, and mycoplasma. At highest risk for PID are women who have had multiple sex partners and failed to use barrier method birth control, such as condoms or diaphragms. Some cases of PID are traced to intrauterine devices or to certain surgical procedures, including abortion and hysterosalpingography. Ironically, the latter procedure, which involves injecting dye into the uterus and fallopian tubes and subjecting them to X-rays, may be performed as part of an infertility diagnostic workup (see Chapter 4).

Like endometriosis, PID may or may not display symptoms. PID symptoms can include pelvic or abdominal pain, fever or chills, spotting between periods, or digestive or urinary problems. Success rates in treating PID and PID-induced adhesions depend on the extent of the damage.

IMMUNOLOGIC INFERTILITY

The body's immune system is dependent in large part on antibodies, which are proteins manufactured by white blood cells to neutralize foreign and presumably hostile proteins called antigens. Antigens are commonly found on viruses, bacteria, and other microorganisms.

In some cases, antibodies attack harmless proteins, causing such problems as arthritis and allergies. What concerns infertility specialists are antibodies that attack antigens on sperm cells. Among infertile couples, this condition exists in about 15 percent to 20 percent of women and 5 percent to 10 percent of men.

There is no known cause of so-called "anti-sperm antibody" production and no definitive cure. However, people with immunologic disorders can often conceive with the help of assisted reproductive technologies.

CERVICAL PROBLEMS

Problems solely with the cervix, the entryway from the vagina to the uterus, are discovered in about 5 percent of infertile women. The role of the cervix is to provide a friendly, nurturing reservoir for sperm. In addition, cervical mucus also filters out "debris": any white blood cells that may be present, and dead and abnormal sperm, as well as prostaglandins, chemicals in the semen that would trigger severe cramps if allowed into the uterus.

A telltale sign of cervical problems is a lack of copious, clear, stretchy mucus around the time of ovulation. Occasionally, the mucus appears normal but contains anti-sperm antibodies. Cervical mucus can be otherwise hostile to sperm if it is too acidic, is harboring an infection or too many white blood cells, or is too dense to allow sperm penetration. Ideally, sperm should be able to live for a couple days in the cervical mucus, which normally nourishes and energizes sperm before releasing them a few at a time into the uterus. This release pattern ups the chances of conception, since intercourse does not always take place precisely when an egg is in position to be fertilized.

Women who have had pieces of their cervix surgically removed suffer a loss of cells responsible for mucus production. This condition is known as a "dry cervix." Cryotherapy, a technique used to kill through freezing cancerous or pre-cancerous cells in the cervix, can result in a dry cervix, as can cauterization—using heat to achieve the same end. Another potential cause is the presence or removal of a tumor, polyp, or other abnormal growth in the cervix. Certain drugs, including the ovulation drug clomiphene citrate, can diminish the quality of cervical mucus (see Chapter 5). Cervical problems can be bypassed through artificial insemination or other assisted reproductive techniques.

Even an otherwise normal cervix can open spontaneously during pregnancy, particularly if the cervix had been weakened owing to repeated stretching with surgical instruments. Some women are simply born with a so-called "incompetent cervix." Unfortunately, the only way to diagnose this relatively rare condition is when it results in a spontaneous abortion. Future problems can be avoided by stitching the cervix closed during the next pregnancy.

POLYCYSTIC OVARIAN DISEASE (PCOD)

Sometimes called Stein-Leventhal syndrome, polycystic ovarian disease is one of the least understood conditions impairing fertility. Afflicting less than 2 percent of infertile women, the disease is spurred by an overproduction of the male hormone testosterone, by the ovaries, and by the adrenal gland. Fat cells convert testosterone to estrogen at an elevated rate, which triggers the pituitary to secrete abnormally high levels of luteinizing hormone. Elevated LH tells the ovaries to produce more testosterone. As a result of this vicious cycle, egg follicles fail to develop completely and instead turn into small ovarian cysts. Infertility, irregular periods, failure to ovulate (anovulation), abnormal hair growth, failure to menstruate, breast secretions, and bad acne all are symptoms of PCOD. The disease is more common among obese women and women with diabetes. There is a variety of treatment approaches to correct PCOD (see Chapter 5).

UTERINE FACTOR

Fibroids—benign tumors known as myomas—inside the uterus are found in about 20 percent of women over age 30 and most frequently occur in women between ages 35 and 45. They are believed to be caused by an abnormal response to estrogen. In many cases, fibroids cause no symptoms at all, especially if the growth is small. Fibroids can range from the size of a pea to the size of a grapefruit or even larger. Fibroids that grow on the outside of the uterus tend not to cause fertility problems.

Inside the uterus is another story. If fibroids are large enough to distort the cavity of the uterus, they can thwart a pregnancy by interfering with a fertilized egg's ability to implant. A fertilized egg will not even reach the uterus if a fibroid is blocking the opening of the fallopian tube. If the egg does implant, a large fibroid anywhere inside the uterus can increase the woman's risk of miscarriage.

If the fibroid grows large enough, it may cause heavy or prolonged menstrual bleeding, pressure on the bladder or bowels, backache or constipation. Surgical removal of fibroids may create another problem: scar tissue.

When a woman suffers repeated miscarriages, her doctor may suspect that something is structurally wrong with her uterus. In most cases, these abnormalities are present at birth and can be corrected through reconstructive or laser surgery.

Again, the surgeon must take great care to keep scarring in the uterus and pelvic cavity at a minimum.

While structural abnormalities are rare, the most common is the presence of a wall, or "septum," dividing the uterine cavity in two. No one knows for sure why some women are born this way. Once the septum is corrected surgically, the woman remains at a slightly higher than average risk for miscarriage, especially if there is more than one fetus.

DES

Almost 35 years ago, obstetricians began prescribing high doses of the drug diethylstilbestrol (DES) to pregnant patients who had a history of miscarriage or who otherwise seemed at high risk for such an event. DES, a type of synthetic estrogen, was banned in the 1970s when researchers noticed a rise in a rare form of vaginal cancer among children exposed to DES in the womb. Many DES daughters and some DES sons were experiencing reproductive difficulties later in life. DES-related problems may include impaired fertility, endometriosis, ectopic pregnancy, and repeated miscarriages. Some DES daughters were born with malformed fallopian tubes that resulted in tubal pregnancies. They may have a uterine cavity shaped like a "T," which can produce miscarriage or premature labor. And DES daughters are more likely to have poor-quality cervical mucus. However, the fact that your mother took DES while she was pregnant with you does not necessarily rule out your chances of becoming pregnant and giving birth.

SMOKING

In the United States, almost 1 in 3 (about 30 percent) women of childbearing age smoke cigarettes. Doctors have known for many years that women smokers tend to have smaller fetuses and shorter gestation periods than non-smokers. Over the last

13 years, several studies have drawn links between smoking and impaired fertility.

One study of pregnancy rates among 678 women, published by the *Journal of the American Medical Association* in 1985, found that smokers were 3.4 times as likely as non-smokers to take more than a year to conceive. Research has shown that, for reasons not fully understood, non-whites seem particularly vulnerable to the fertility-impairing effects of smoking.

Smokers who do become pregnant have almost a twofold increase in miscarriage rates (14.4–27 percent) compared with the general population (12–15 percent). For one thing, smoking is believed to reduce estrogen levels. Smokers also risk shortening their reproductive life. Women who smoke a half-pack of cigarettes a day undergo menopause an average of one year earlier than non-smokers. Those who smoke a pack a day or more will, on average, be menopausal two years earlier. These data have led researchers to conclude that women who smoke may irreversibly be reducing their store of eggs and possibly be diminishing the quality of their remaining eggs.

Fallopian tubes don't escape the deleterious effects of cigarette smoke, either. Smokers appear to be three times more likely to have an ectopic pregnancy, according to the World Health Organization. One reason may be that smoking impairs the tubes' ability to carry an egg toward the uterus. Smoking also suppresses the immune system, making smokers more susceptible to sexually transmitted diseases, which are associated with ectopic pregnancy and other fertility problems.

If you're still not convinced, consider these data from a 1984–89 study conducted by H. Anthony Pattison, M.D., and colleagues at Alberta Children's Hospital in Calgary, Alberta, Canada, comparing in-vitro fertilization outcomes where 124 of the women smoked and 236 did not. With an overall per-cycle pregnancy rate of 19.2 percent, 21.2 percent of non-smokers got pregnant compared with only 15.3 percent of smokers. What's worse, the incidence of miscarriage was 18.9 percent in non-smokers and a whopping 42.1 percent in smokers.

RECURRENT MISCARRIAGE

As in infertility, there are many potential causes for repeated miscarriage, not the least of which is age. Since the optimal time for having children is between ages 20 and 34, miscarriage is more likely among older women. Doctors generally do not suspect a chronic problem—and thus do not order diagnostic testing—until after the second or third miscarriage.

About 50 percent to 60 percent of first-trimester miscarriages occur when the fetus has a chromosomal abnormality. Miscarriage due to a genetic abnormality in either the mother or the father occurs only about 8 percent of the time. Testing the tissue of a miscarried fetus uncovers only a small percentage of those pregnancies lost because of genetic problems. If the tissue typing is abnormal, nothing can be done to lessen the chance of a recurrence. An amniocentesis during any subsequent pregnancy would be recommended.

The risk of spontaneous abortion after three successive miscarriages is about 30 percent to 50 percent. The chance of a successful live birth after three consecutive miscarriages without a live birth is 40 percent to 50 percent, while the chance of a successful live birth following one abnormal pregnancy is about 70 percent.

In 10 percent to 15 percent of miscarriages, a uterine or cervical abnormality is discovered. Miscarriage also has been linked to a hyperactive or underactive thyroid gland, a condition that usually can be treated with hormonal supplements.

Research has suggested that a minority of women may be losing pregnancies because their immune system is rejecting the fetus. There is much debate in this area, however. There are no reliable tests to detect this form of immunologic miscarriage and no approved therapy to prevent it.

If the mother's immune system is producing so-called "anti-phospholipid" antibodies, which attack clotting components in the blood, this also can cause enough fetal harm to trigger a miscarriage. Some doctors prescribe aspirin and prednisone (a steroid) in an attempt to combat this condition.

Unfortunately, there is no clear cause in about 40 percent of women who have recurrent miscarriage.

DEFECTIVE EGGS

The newest explanation for infertility is lack of fertilization because of defective eggs. The reasons a woman of childbearing age would have defective eggs are unclear. Unfortunately, diagnosis of this rare condition cannot occur until the couple's first attempt at in-vitro fertilization. IVF is considered too costly and complicated to perform for the sole purpose of diagnosis. When it is attempted for therapeutic reasons, about 13 percent to 16 percent of IVF attempts will result in no fertilization. But impaired egg quality is to blame in only some of these cases, researchers surmise. The only possible solutions would be donor eggs or micromanipulation of the eggs, according to Yossef Ezra, M.D., and colleagues at Hadassah University Hospital in Jerusalem.

WHAT CAN GO WRONG IN MEN?

While female infertility usually has nothing to do with the quality of a woman's eggs, male infertility almost always manifests in a diminished quality or quantity of sperm. Normal semen contains at least 20 million sperm cells per milliliter (ml), or 150 million to 200 million sperm per ejaculation.

Normally, at least half those sperm are "motile," or moving, in a progressive direction, not wandering aimlessly or swimming in circles. The motility rate should be more or less constant over the next two to four hours. The semen should be virtually free of white blood cells. At least 40 to 50 percent should be normally shaped. Generally speaking, it is better for fertility to have a low sperm count but good sperm quality than the other way around.

When determining whether to use the husband's sperm for an artificial insemination, specialists look for a minimum volume of 1 to 2 ml of semen with 20 million sperm per ml. About 40 percent of the sperm should be motile, and at least 50 percent of the sperm cells should be normal.

Even if a man's sperm count is below average, the woman may become pregnant with relative ease if she is extremely fertile.

VARICOCELE

One potential cause of abnormal sperm is a varicocele, which is actually an enlarged vein, also known as a varicose vein—like the kind that forms blue lines on the legs of some older adults. However, a varicocele is too deep to be seen on the skin and is usually found just above the left testicle in one or more of the primary vessels that carry blood from the groin back to the heart. While about 8 percent of the male population has a varicocele, it doesn't always result in infertility. A varicocele is at least twice as common among infertile men, however, being diagnosed in 20 to 30 percent of cases. There are no symptoms.

No one knows why a varicocele forms or exactly how a varicocele impairs fertility, although most experts believe that it makes the temperature inside the testicles too high for normal sperm development to occur. Sperm need a relatively cool environment to form properly; that's why the testicles hang outside the body.

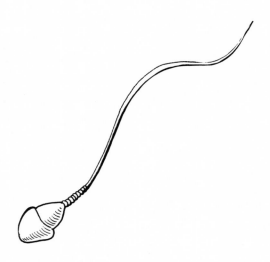

FIGURE 4   A normally formed sperm.

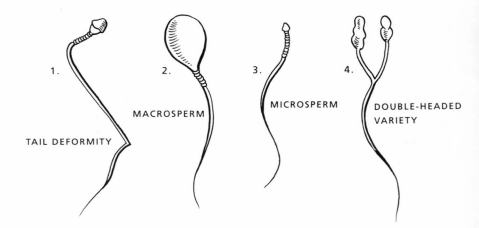

FIGURE 5   Various abnormal sperm forms commonly seen: 1. Tail deformity; 2. Macrosperm; 3. Microsperm; 4. Double-headed variety.

A physician may suspect a varicocele if the semen has a low sperm concentration and contains a large proportion of dead and sluggish sperm. In particular, sperm with abnormally small, tapered heads often indicate a varicocele is present. Microsurgery to tie off the varicocele may improve sperm quality and quantity in about 50 percent to 70 percent of cases. However, only 30 percent to 40 percent of these men will ultimately impregnate their wives, some studies suggest. And it is impossible to predict who will respond to surgery and who will not. Furthermore, the size of the varicocele seems to have no bearing on the outcome of surgery.

FERTILE IDEA

While there is no direct evidence that this works, some practitioners advise male patients with fertility problems to wear boxer shorts instead of tight-fitting underwear. Tight underwear presses testicles close to the body, raising the temperature of the testicles and creating a less-than-ideal environment for healthy sperm production. Excessive or prolonged physical activity can also raise the temperature inside the testicles.

BLOCKAGES

Inside the testicles lies an intricate network of ducts, or tunnels, through which sperm travel as they mature. If one or more of these ducts get blocked because of infection (including sexually transmitted disease), surgical scarring, or trauma, sperm can be prevented from exiting the penis. If there is an active infection, there will be numerous white blood cells in the semen.

HORMONAL IMBALANCE

In a minority of cases, the pituitary gland fails to secrete sufficient luteinizing hormone or follicle-stimulating hormone needed to stimulate the testicles to produce sperm. A growth in the pituitary is one possible explanation for this condition.

ANTI-SPERM ANTIBODIES

Just as a woman can be "allergic" to her husband's sperm, a man may form antibodies against his own sperm. The condition is rare, and its cause is unknown. Doctors suspect the presence of anti-sperm antibodies when sperm clump together.

SEXUAL DYSFUNCTION

If a man is unable to achieve an erection or ejaculate, he obviously cannot begin to deliver his sperm to his wife's egg. This condition does not necessarily mean that there is something wrong with his sperm or that it can't be extracted and used for in-vitro fertilization.

RETROGRADE EJACULATION

In cases of retrograde ejaculation, the semen backs up through the urethra into the bladder. It is sometimes possible to harvest healthy sperm from urine and use it in artificial insemination.

ILLNESS

A variety of illnesses can diminish the body's ability to produce sperm. Since it takes about three months for sperm to fully mature, it usually takes that long for sperm counts to bounce back to normal after a bout with the flu. Certain other illnesses can cause permanent infertility. About 50 percent of men who contract the mumps after puberty suffer irreparable damage to the testicles and wind up with a very low sperm count or no sperm at all. Men with diabetes mellitus also are susceptible to fertility problems. Men who must undergo cancer chemotherapy or radiation but still hope to father children someday can bank their sperm before treatment begins.

AGENT ORANGE

Approximately 500,000 men were exposed to the powerful defoliant Agent Orange during the Vietnam War. Twenty years later, some of these veterans were having reproductive problems. In late 1992, researchers at Rutgers University reported that many of the 97 Vietnam veterans they had been studying had low sperm counts and high numbers of deformed and poor-swimming sperm. In the opinion of Rutgers biochemist Peter Kahn, a larger study is needed to ascertain any cause and effect between fertility impairment and exposure to dioxin, a highly toxic chemical found in Agent Orange.

WHAT CAN GO WRONG IN BOTH PARTNERS?

As mentioned previously, infertility stems from both a male and a female factor in about 20 percent of couples who seek treatment. A bacterial infection can be passed back and forth during intercourse, impairing both partners' reproductive capacities. The wife may have endometriosis, and her husband may have anti-sperm antibodies. A wife may have a dry cervix and irregular periods, and her husband may have a varicocele. There are countless possible combinations.

Additionally, exposure to certain substances can affect both male and female gametes (sperm and egg cells) as well as hormonal balances in both sexes.

TOXIC EXPOSURES

Our world is awash in tens of thousands of toxic chemicals, both man-made and natural. We breathe these toxins, eat them in the form of pesticides on food and hormones in meat, and we work around them in our manufacturing plants. Over the last 25 years, the Food and Drug Administration and the Environmental Protection Agency have adopted regulations requiring medications, food additives, pesticides, and other chemicals to be tested for reproductive toxicity. These tests are generally done on animals. Despite these regulations, there is much that we don't know about toxins and their potential impact on human reproduction.

According to the research that has been done, timing of a toxic exposure is important when looking at health effects. A onetime toxic exposure may produce subtle changes in a man's hormonal output, resulting in a temporary drop in sperm count. That same exposure in a woman may damage some of her eggs, or "profoundly influence ovarian or uterine physiology," concluded Betts Field, Ph.D., and colleagues at Duke University after reviewing relevant studies for an article in the February 1990 issue of *Seminars in Reproductive Endocrinology*. "Toxins may affect the reproductive system during adulthood, but most effects seem to be reversible when exposure ends," their article states.

FERTILE IDEA

If you work near solvents, such as those used in the computer-manufacturing industry, around the time you are trying to conceive, you may want to consider changing jobs, or jobsites, temporarily at least. Certain solvents are believed to impair fertility and fecundity.

Occupational exposure to high levels of nitrous oxide—the "laughing gas" used in up to half of all dental offices—also may adversely affect a woman's ability to become pregnant, according to Andrew S. Rowland, Ph.D., and colleagues at the National Institute of Environmental Health Sciences. That conclusion was reached after extensive interviews with almost 500 dental assistants in California. The study, published in the October 1, 1992, issue of the *New England Journal of Medicine,* found that dental workers exposed to nitrous oxide took 32 months to conceive, on average, compared with an average of six months for women who were not exposed to the gas. The reason for this phenomenon was unclear.

Researchers recommend that if you are one of the more than 270,000 female dentists, dental assistants, and hygienists working in this country, be sure your office has "scavenging" equipment, which captures stray nitrous oxide. And certainly don't inhale the gas for recreational purposes. Dental patients exposed to laughing gas on occasion are not at risk.

Other substances that appear to impair reproduction are DDT and chlorinated hydrocarbons. Dr. Field states that these substances may affect implantation of fertilized eggs in animals, probably because the chemicals cause an estrogen imbalance. If you work around chemicals, ask your employer for a list of compounds you are exposed to and give this list to your doctor.

Providing your doctor with an accurate family history is another important step in tracking down fertility problems that may stem from toxic exposures. Exposure in the womb to certain agents, such as DES, can damage a male's reproductive tract as well as a female's.

SUBSTANCE ABUSE

"Although the research on the reproductive effects of substance abuse is far from complete, the studies show potentially serious risks to reproduction and fertility," according to Carol Grace Smith, Ph.D., of the University of Texas Health Science Center, and Michael Smith, M.D., of the Medical College of Georgia. The heavier the abuse, the graver the risk, they say.

As many as 10 percent of people in childbearing years are alcoholics, and about 30 percent of women in their late teens and early 20s use marijuana. Alcohol can result in abnormal sperm—either short-term or long-term, depending on the extent of abuse. Chronic alcoholism has been linked to infertility and menstrual disorders in women.

Delta-9-tetrahydrocannabinol (THC), the primary psychoactive ingredient in marijuana, inhibits the secretion of reproductive hormones, including LH and FSH, in women. This can result in irregular periods. THC exposure in early pregnancy may raise the miscarriage risk, but the data are somewhat contradictory in this area.

In men, THC has been shown to lower testosterone output. One study looked at men who smoked pot for four weeks and then abstained. Two weeks later, their sperm counts dropped significantly. "It is clear," the researchers say, "that marijuana use should be considered as a factor that may contribute to unexplained infertility in men."

While there are no published studies of the possible effects of cocaine on reproductive hormones, that drug has been linked to serious complications in pregnancy, including an increased rate of spontaneous abortion in the first trimester, the same researchers point out. Heroin has been shown to decrease male fertility while causing male sex organs to atrophy.

POOR TIMING

Even if neither spouse has a fertility problem, pregnancy will not occur if intercourse is poorly timed. Have intercourse every other day to keep sperm count at optimal levels. Counting the first day of your period as day 1, be sure to have intercourse between days 9 and 15 of the menstrual cycle, based on a 28-day cycle. If your cycle is longer or shorter, make sure to have intercourse every other day in the middle of your cycle. (More frequent intercourse will not allow sperm sufficient time to replenish.) Granted, following this pattern diminishes spontaneity and romance. But, for now, planned intercourse is vital in order to reach your immediate goal: becoming parents.

CHAPTER 3

FINDING A DOCTOR

If you were searching for an internist or a dentist, you could ask any friend or co-worker for a recommendation. But when you're looking for an infertility specialist or IVF clinic, the search can be quite a challenge.

Finding a qualified infertility doctor or fertility clinic is a crucial step in your journey toward pregnancy. Ideally, your physician will be experienced and competent, have a caring bedside manner, have helped many women become pregnant and have babies, listen and communicate effectively, and practice within a reasonable distance of your home. For Sherry, the gynecologist she had been seeing for years seemed to fit the bill. Or so she thought.

Sherry had been a patient of Dr. Klein's for six years when she and Jeff got married. Because they were in their early 30s and established in their professions, Sherry and Jeff began trying to have a baby almost immediately. After six months passed with no pregnancy, Dr. Klein renewed his advice to "relax" and to have intercourse every other day. Sherry and Jeff followed his words diligently. After all, Dr. Klein listed infertility in the yellow pages and on his business card as one of his specialties. When another six months passed with no pregnancy, Dr. Klein ordered a semen analysis for Jeff. He also ordered an X-ray test of Sherry's fallopian tubes, and a month later performed a laparoscopy to examine her reproductive organs.

When none of those tests turned up any abnormalities, Dr.

Klein told Sherry to come in for a $75 consultation. At the consultation, which was repeatedly interrupted by a ringing telephone and nurses popping their heads into his office, Dr. Klein offered to refer Sherry to an infertility specialist.

"But I thought that *you* specialized in infertility," Sherry said.

"Infertility testing, not treatment," Dr. Klein responded.

He wrote down a name of a doctor who practiced three counties away—at least an hour's drive, without traffic, from Sherry and Jeff's house. Sherry wondered why Dr. Klein hadn't simply given her the name over the phone.

"But I understand that infertility treatment involves dozens of visits," Sherry protested. "How can I relax if I have to spend two hours in a car fighting traffic every time I need to see the doctor? Don't you know of anyone closer who can help us?"

"No, there's no one nearby who's good enough," Dr. Klein said. "This doctor gets results."

Feeling almost betrayed by a doctor she had thought could treat her fertility problem, Sherry left Dr. Klein's office despondent. Seeing no other choice, she called the specialist Dr. Klein referred her to, only to learn there was a two-month wait for an appointment. She made one and bided her time.

A couple of weeks later, Sherry read in her local newspaper about a physician, Dr. Lehigh, in the next town who had quietly specialized in infertility diagnosis and treatment for almost 20 years. Two of the hundreds of women who had become pregnant under Dr. Lehigh's care were quoted in the article. Also mentioned was the formation of a local support group for couples experiencing infertility.

Sherry joined the support group and called Dr. Lehigh's office almost immediately. To her delight, she was able to get an appointment two weeks later. While Dr. Lehigh maintained a bustling OB–GYN practice, he also performed artificial inseminations in his office, was hooked into a sperm bank, and served as a satellite clinic for a full-scale infertility treatment center at a nearby teaching hospital.

The moral of Sherry's story is "buyer beware." While the number of bona fide doctors and clinics specializing in infertility has risen dramatically in recent years, the number of physicians like Dr. Klein who exaggerate the extent of their infertility practice has probably risen even higher. If your gynecologist lists "infertility" on his or her shingle, ask exactly what that means. Is the physician specially trained in reproductive endocrinology? Does he or she offer hormonal testing? Drug therapy? Artificial inseminations? In-vitro fertilizations and related procedures?

While there's nothing wrong with having your regular gynecologist begin some diagnostic tests, know his or her limits from the onset. To save time, especially if you're in your mid-30s or older, you may want to find a doctor or clinic offering a whole range of infertility services as soon as you suspect a fertility problem.

Generally, though, infertility is not suspected unless you've tried and failed to become pregnant for at least 12 months. Some doctors are willing to begin a diagnostic workup after six months, particularly if the woman is over 34 years old. However, there is no reason to wait even six months before seeking help if you know you've had pelvic inflammatory disease, prenatal DES exposure, endometriosis, or have had an ovary removed or surgery on your tubes, or if your husband is already aware that his sperm count is abnormally low.

Many couples can obtain a referral to a fertility specialist through the wife's gynecologist or the family's internist. Here are some other ways to learn the names of fertility specialists in your area:

- Ask the American Fertility Society for a roster of members in your region. The society's address and phone number can be found in the Resources section at the end of this book. The organization, which sets scientifically backed standards for practice, also can provide you with the names and addresses of IVF centers in your state. You can be assured that society members have advanced training in infertility diagnosis and treatment and receive medical journals designed to keep them abreast of developments in their field.

- Call or write the national Resolve office for a list of support groups near your home. Resolve's address and phone number also are listed in the Resources section. Most Resolve members have extensive experience with the infertility doctors and can steer you in the right direction.

- Get in touch with the nearest large hospital to learn whether it has a fertility clinic. Teaching hospitals, particularly ones in metropolitan areas, are most likely to offer infertility services. Before becoming a patient there, make sure they follow the standards set by the American Fertility Society and the Society for Advanced Reproductive Technology.

- If you have a friend or acquaintance who benefited from a local infertility doctor, ask for a recommendation.

- If you belong to a managed care system, such as a health-maintenance organization (HMO) or a preferred-provider organization (PPO), your options are somewhat limited. If there's no infertility specialist in the group, ask to be referred to one.

Generally, infertility specialists are gynecologists, who have received additional training in reproductive endocrinology and infertility, or reproductive endocrinologists. If you have irregular periods or another reason to suspect a hormonal imbalance, select a reproductive endocrinologist. These doctors have advanced training in measuring various hormone levels in your blood at different times in your cycle, interpreting that information correctly, and prescribing a remedy. If your problem is a male factor, a urologist with extensive infertility experience is apt to know the laboratory with the best reputation for conducting an accurate and detailed semen analysis. A urologist specializing in male infertility is also experienced in performing surgery aimed at correcting male-factor problems.

If you live in a rural area, your choices might be limited to one specialist. If you live in a more densely populated region, you may end up with a list of three or four infertility specialists who may or may not work in an IVF clinic. The next step is interviewing these physicians and probing their backgrounds— just as you would do with a job applicant if you were a business owner. Unfortunately, in this largely unregulated industry, it is not unheard of for doctors to inflate their success rates. When you ask about the doctor's track record, find out what percentage of his or her infertility cases resulted in live births. To learn whether the doctor has ever been sanctioned or disciplined for professional misconduct, call your county or state board of medical examiners, the state agency that licenses the medical profession.

In its 1990 report, the American Fertility Society's ethics committee said that prospective patients should be informed of the guidelines the clinic follows to help women get pregnant. "Clinics offering untried technologies should disclose this fact," the committee wrote. "Prospective patients should be fully aware of the risks and benefits of the proposed procedures."

The committee further recommends that patients be told of the nature of the organization offering infertility services: "whether it is part of an academic center, a private practice, a commercial organization, etc."

Your investigation process need not entail a costly consultation with each physician. Often, the doctor or a receptionist can answer most of your questions over the phone. Take notes, and judge each doctor based on *all* the answers together.

Here are some questions to ask:

- Are you board certified in obstetrics and gynecology?
- Have you completed a fellowship in reproductive endocrinology?
- Are you a member of the American Fertility Society? The Society for Advanced Reproductive Technology?
- How long have you been in infertility practice?
- What do the various procedures cost? Will you work directly with my health-insurance company to obtain reimbursement, or must I pay at the time of treatment and then file my own claims?
- How many infertility patients do you have currently? Is there a waiting list for an appointment?
- Do you also treat obstetrical patients? If so, do you have a separate waiting area for infertility patients? (You may find it uncomfortable to sit in a waiting room filled with pregnant women.)
- Do you offer a full range of diagnostic testing?
- Do you have an ultrasound machine on site? (Frequent ultrasound scans of the ovaries are an integral part of most infertility treatments. If you must travel to a hospital each time you need a scan, treatment through this doctor will be needlessly time-consuming.)
- Do you offer artificial inseminations? Are you willing to perform an insemination on a weekend or holiday, if necessary? (As you will see in Chapter 6, proper timing of infertility treatments is critical.)
- What kinds of surgical treatments do you offer?
- Do you perform assisted reproductive technologies such as in-vitro fertilization, GIFT, and ZIFT? (See Chapter 6.)
- Can you help me obtain donor sperm, donor eggs, or donor embryos through your office if I should need to go this route? Does the sperm bank you use employ a

director who has been trained by the American Association of Tissue Banks?

- What are your pregnancy and take-home baby rates for couples with our particular problem (if your problem has already been diagnosed)? Don't ask simply for the doctor's "success rate" without specifying what you mean by "success." The pregnancy rate will always be higher than the take-home baby rate.
- What are your pregnancy and take-home baby rates for various procedures, and how do your numbers compare with national success rates?
- Do you have a psychologist, social worker, or nurse on staff who can support me emotionally should I need it? Or can you refer me to an outside counselor or support group?
- How would you describe your bedside manner? Of course, this question is best answered during a face-to-face meeting. Consider whether the doctor makes you feel calm or tense. Does he or she seem happy or reluctant to answer your questions? Does the doctor give you undivided attention? Does he or she speak in laymen's terms or "medicalese?" Does the doctor seem sympathetic to your plight, or do you walk out of the meeting feeling like just another medical challenge?
- (If the clinic is located a long distance from your home . . .) Could you refer me to a local physician who can get me started on ovulation drugs before I travel to you for an insemination or IVF procedure?

While evaluating each physician or clinic, it's important to follow your instincts. For example, if a Dr. ABC has been in private infertility practice for only a year but has already achieved several pregnancies, and she is also compassionate and a good listener, you may feel comfortable enough to put yourself under her care. If Dr. XYZ has been in practice 15 years, has an average success rate, but is demeaning during your interview and uses medical jargon you don't understand, you may want to go elsewhere.

Choose your doctor or clinic wisely. After all, you may be in treatment for some time to come.

CHAPTER 4

DIAGNOSING INFERTILITY

There may be a strong temptation to blame yourself for the difficulty you are having getting pregnant or staying pregnant. While your reproductive system may be malfunctioning, there's an equally strong chance that something is awry with your husband's. It is also possible, as is true in as many as 20 percent of cases, that the problem is shared.

Regardless of the cause or causes, try to remember that your sensuality and femininity and your husband's masculinity need not be threatened by your dilemma. By remembering this, you will have an easier time keeping your self-esteem intact as you begin the largely unpleasant process of infertility diagnosis. This painstaking endeavor is unavoidable if you are to begin to take charge of your situation and work to turn it around.

Expect to be poked, prodded, scraped, stuck with needles, injected with dye, explored with surgical instruments, and to experience some embarrassment during the diagnostic phase. Also expect to be charged anywhere from $500 to $2,000 or more for these tests, depending on your doctor, where you live, and the complexity of your problem. The good news is that, with careful planning, you can often obtain a diagnosis in as little as a month or two.

As you learned in Chapter 2, there are many potential causes of infertility. It therefore is important that both you and your husband be tested. Doctors usually test the male's semen first, since it is far simpler and less costly to evaluate sperm than it is to diagnose the cause of female infertility. Some health insurers will deny coverage of diagnostic tests for the female partner if they are ordered before results of the male partner's semen analysis are known.

Even after undergoing a battery of tests, however, about 15 of every 100 infertile couples will discover no apparent cause of their infertility. Although a diagnosis of unknown causes is frustrating, it does not necessarily mean the couple will not respond to treatment resulting in a pregnancy.

DIAGNOSING MALE INFERTILITY

MEDICAL HISTORY

Before ordering a semen analysis, the infertility specialist will want to know much about your husband's background and medical history. He must disclose: diseases, including any bouts with sexually transmitted diseases; hospitalizations and surgeries; use of drugs, both prescription and illicit; accidents or trauma involving the genitals; past and present medical problems; his parents' health history, including whether his mother took DES while she was pregnant with him; use of tobacco (including smokeless brands); alcohol consumption; impotence or other sexual problems; and exposure to Agent Orange or other hazardous substances.

Candor is key. Without an accurate and complete medical history, the physician may miss an important diagnostic clue.

Remind your husband that a doctor-patient relationship is completely private, so if he is using marijuana, for instance, the doctor cannot report him to the police.

PHYSICAL EXAMINATION

A urologist or family physician will make note of your husband's sexual development and distribution of body hair, since abnormalities can indicate a possible hormonal imbalance. The doctor will then look for surgical scars and examine his penis, taking a culture of any discharge that might be present. He also will examine the testicles for abnormalities.

SEMEN ANALYSIS

The first time your husband is asked to ejaculate into a plastic cup may be traumatic for him. He might as well get used to it, though, since the first time won't be his last. At least three or four semen analyses over a course of two months are usually ordered, for many factors can temporarily depress sperm counts (see Chapter 2). If you wind up using any of the assisted reproductive technologies described later in this book, ejaculating into a plastic cup will become routine for your husband. Your doctor or the laboratory performing the analysis can provide him with a supply of sterile cups.

Your husband should refrain from intercourse and masturbation for about 48 hours before producing the sample to be analyzed. This gives his body enough time to replenish the sperm. Some labs do semen analyses only during certain hours or certain days of the week. It's therefore important to make an appointment with the lab at least a week in advance.

FERTILE IDEA

If you live within 60 minutes of the lab, your husband can produce the semen sample at home. He should place the cup containing the semen in a shirt pocket to keep it close to body temperature en route to the lab. If the sample gets too cold, a portion of the sperm cells will die, skewing the accuracy of the analysis. If you live farther away, be sure the lab has a room designated for semen collection. If the lab has no such room, you should suspect that semen analyses are not performed there routinely and the results might be incomplete or inaccurate. If the lab has a designated room, your husband may wish to bring along an X-rated magazine. Or you can ask to accompany him.

Once the semen sample has been obtained, the lab technician will begin the analysis within the hour. Semen, which, as noted earlier, normally takes on a jelly-like consistency soon after ejaculation, should liquify within a half-hour. If it doesn't, the doctor may suspect that your husband lacks seminal vesicles or a vas deferens.

Semen volume should also be measured, since too much or too little semen can contribute to infertility. Normally, a man ejaculates between 2 and 4 milliliters of semen. Normal semen also gives off a pungent odor after 20 minutes or so. If the odor is absent, there may be a dysfunctioning prostate gland at fault. If the semen is white or yellow instead of the normal whitish-gray, there may be too many white blood cells in it, indicating an infection. Infection of the sexual organs also may be suspected if the semen's pH value is above 8, meaning it is too alkaline.

Using a specially equipped microscope, the technician will count the number of live, dead, and malformed sperm. The technician also will assess whether the sperm are swimming in a progressive fashion. The presence of "debris," such as white blood cells, should be noted on the lab report, as well.

VARICOCELE STUDY

If the sperm count is too low and there are many sperm with abnormally small heads, the doctor may suspect the presence of a varicose vein, or varicocele, usually above the left testicle. Normally, valves inside veins prevent the blood from flowing backward. Because the valves in a vein affected by a varicocele are faulty, blood pools in the area. This pooling is thought to raise the temperature inside the testicles and adversely affect sperm development.

A varicocele can often be detected with a stethoscope by a urologist or an experienced internist. If the doctor hears blood flowing through a varicocele, he may order an ultrasound scan to confirm the diagnosis, assess its size, and pinpoint its location.

HORMONAL TESTS

If the man has an extremely low sperm count or no sperm at all, a series of endocrine studies should be ordered. These blood tests measure levels of thyroid-stimulating hormone, testosterone, follicle-stimulating hormone, luteinizing hormone, and prolactin.

ANTI-SPERM ANTIBODY TEST

If the sperm seem to have difficulty penetrating the cervical mucus (see post-coital test below), or the sperm cells clump together, the doctor may order an anti-sperm antibody test. Anti-sperm antibodies, which attack a man's own sperm, are most commonly detected with an "immunobead test." In this test, sperm are mixed with microscopic beads that have antibodies attached to them. Anti-sperm antibodies are diagnosed if at least 10 percent of the sperm adhere to the beads. Immunobeads also can be used to test a woman's cervical mucus and serum for the presence of anti-sperm antibodies.

PENETRATION TESTS

Semen is placed into a long tube containing either egg whites or vaginal mucus taken from a cow. By measuring how far up the tube the sperm can swim, doctors estimate the sperm's ability to penetrate human cervical mucus. About 80 percent of men scoring well on a sperm-penetration test will do well with in-vitro fertilization; 80 percent who score poorly are unable to produce sperm capable of fertilizing an egg. Similarly, sperm's ability to penetrate a hamster egg is a fair indicator—although no guarantee—of whether it can penetrate a human egg. Both the mucus and the hamster egg tests may be ordered late in the workup, usually in anticipation of IVF.

TESTICULAR BIOPSY

Another test offered late in the workup, if at all, is a biopsy of testicular tissue. By examining testicular tissue microscopically, the doctor may be able to find inflammation or scar tissue in the tubules. A biopsy also enables the doctor to track the maturation process of the sperm.

FRUCTOSE TEST

If your husband's semen contains no sperm at all, a condition known as "azoospermia," the doctor will probably order a fructose test. Fructose, a type of sugar, should be present in semen. If it is not, it could mean there is a blockage in the ductal system.

DIAGNOSING FEMALE INFERTILITY

From day 1 of his workup, your husband must rely on doctors and lab technicians. You, on the other hand, can take a number of steps independently of your doctor to pave the path toward your own diagnosis.

TEMPERATURE CHART

As soon as you decide to start a family, begin charting your basal (or resting) body temperature every morning. Basal body temperature (BBT) charts are available from gynecologists. Charts also come with thermometers designed for this purpose. Mercury and digital thermometers are both accurate, although the new digital thermometers work more quickly and are easier to read. A blank chart for you to photocopy appears later in this chapter, along with charts showing examples of normal and abnormal temperature readings for you to use as a guide.

Begin taking your temperature on day 1, which is the first day of your period. Take your temperature orally, rectally, or vaginally (chose one method and be consistent) every morning before getting out of bed or stirring in any way. Normally, your temperature rises .5 to 1 point, fairly abruptly, around the time of ovulation. Your temperature should fall slightly just before menstruation. Normal body temperatures vary slightly from person to person, and it is the relative changes within an individual's daily temperature reading that are important.

A record of the rises and falls of your temperature over two or three menstrual cycles enables your doctor to deduce quickly whether ovulation is probably occurring. If your temperature is more or less the same throughout your cycle, chances are you're not releasing an egg. If your temperature remains elevated for more than two weeks after ovulation, conception may have occurred.

In addition to recording your temperature, you should also indicate on the charts when you have intercourse, when your period begins and ends, what days you are ill, and what days you take any medication (illness and drugs can affect body temperature). If you are among the 25 percent of women who experience pain on one side of your abdomen during ovulation, note this occurrence on your charts, as well.

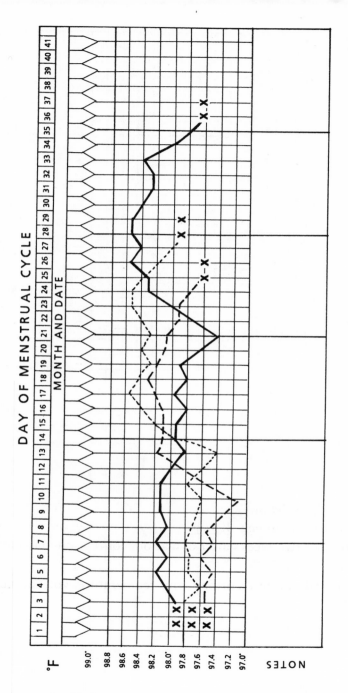

FIGURE 6 Basal body temperature (BBT) chart showing three normal patterns.

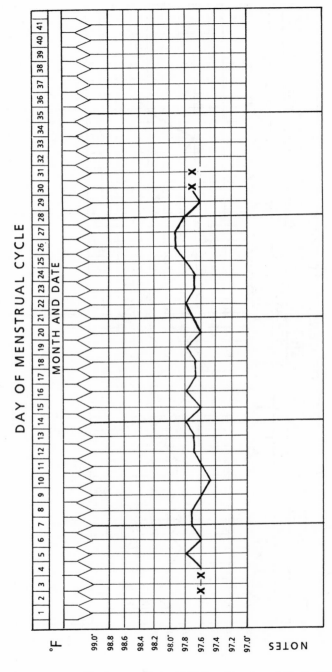

FIGURE 7 Basal body temperature (BBT) chart showing a lack of ovulation.

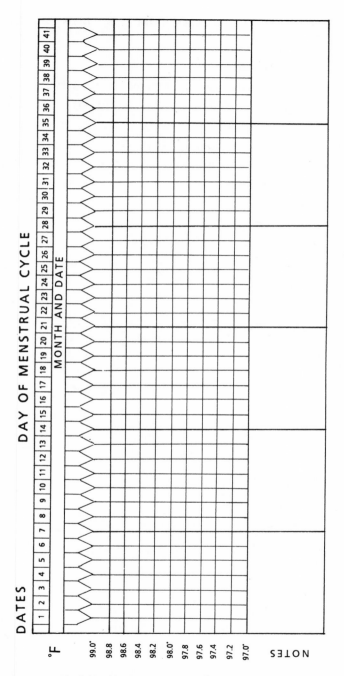

FIGURE 8 Blank basal body temperature (BBT) chart for the reader's use. Copy this chart and use it to keep track of your own temperature.

MUCUS CHANGES

To aid sperm in its journey, mucus in the cervix normally grows more plentiful, clear, and elastic, similar to the consistency of an egg white, just prior to and during ovulation—the time when you are most likely to become pregnant. Cervical mucus is either absent or more sticky and opaque during other times of the month. Noticing your mucus changes can help you to better time intercourse.

HOME OVULATION-PREDICTOR KITS

Some half-dozen kits are available, without prescription, at drugstores. Ranging in price from about $20 to $70, these kits are designed to test urine for a luteinizing hormone (LH) surge. The LH surge triggers the egg to be released from its follicle (ovulation). Research has shown that these home test kits are reliable. Begin testing your urine around day 9 and continue testing until a positive result occurs.

Most ovulation kits come with a five-day supply of testers, and some kits are more complicated than others. In most cases, the user puts her urine in contact with a chemically treated strip or pours urine into a chemically treated test tube and looks for a telltale color change. Because different brands of ovulation-detection kits vary by method, speed, and sensitivity, follow the instructions carefully. The instructions give you a window of time to have intercourse—usually 24 to 48 hours—after a positive test result. The test kits also are helpful for couples undergoing artificial inseminations.

Anytime you notice a mucus change or your home test indicates an LH surge, note it on your temperature chart. As you can see, these charts—if kept diligently as soon as you begin your pregnancy quest—encapsulate a tremendous amount of information. By showing them to your infertility specialist early on, you may be cutting months off the time it takes to reach a diagnosis.

DIAGNOSTIC WORKUP UNDER A DOCTOR'S CARE

While it's helpful to do what you can on your own, there are important diagnostic tests only your doctor can order. How many tests you will undergo and in which order will depend largely on your particular situation.

MEDICAL HISTORY

Before ordering any diagnostic tests, your doctor should obtain a complete medical history, including: length of marriage; length of infertility; frequency of intercourse; past illnesses and diseases (sexually transmitted diseases and others); hospitalizations and surgeries, particularly gynecological or other pelvic region surgery; drug use (prescription and illicit); medical problems past and present, including endometriosis, diabetes, and thyroid disease; family health history, including whether your mother used DES while she was pregnant with you; prior pregnancies, miscarriages, abortions; birth-control history, including use of IUDs and oral contraceptives; menstrual history (age of onset, length of cycle, regularity, nature of flow); tobacco and alcohol use; toxic exposures; height, weight, and level of physical activity.

PHYSICAL EXAMINATION

In search for possible hormonal imbalances, the doctor will examine your thyroid gland and notice the distribution of facial and body hair as well as any milky discharge from your nipples (there should be no discharge in a non-pregnant, non-lactating woman). During a pelvic exam, the doctor will look for growths or other irregularities in your vagina and cervix and examine your cervix for infection or narrowing.

CULTURES AND BLOOD TESTS

During the pelvic exam, a vaginal culture should be taken to test for the presence of harmful organisms. The doctor also should notice whether the consistency of your cervical mucus is appropriate for the day of the cycle you are in.

If the physical exam and BBT charts suggest a hormonal imbalance, more extensive blood testing at various times during your menstrual cycle should be ordered. Levels of luteinizing hormone (LH); follicle-stimulating hormone (FSH); estradiol (a form of estrogen); prolactin, testosterone, progesterone and thyroid-stimulating hormone (TSH) can all be measured through blood tests.

ENDOMETRIAL BIOPSY

If your doctor suspects a luteal phase defect, she may perform an endometrial biopsy. A defect in the luteal phase—the second half of your menstrual cycle—is usually a result of a progesterone deficiency. Without sufficient progesterone, the uterine lining, or endometrium, will be too thin to allow a fertilized egg to implant and grow.

The biopsy is usually done in the doctor's office on day 26 or 27 of your cycle. The procedure may cause brief cramping and pain, so you may want to request a Motrin or an Anaprox beforehand. To perform the biopsy, the doctor will insert a sterile catheter through your vagina and cervix and into your uterus in order to scrape out a small amount of endometrial tissue. Examining the tissue under a microscope, a pathologist can determine what day of your cycle the tissue corresponds to by looking at its density and composition. If you are two days away from your period but the endometrium is only 10 days old, you will probably be diagnosed with a luteal phase defect. If you tried to become pregnant earlier that cycle, take a pregnancy test prior to the biopsy; this causes a miscarriage in about 1 in 1,000 cases. Other risks include infection and bleeding.

POST-COITAL TEST (PCT)

This painless, although somewhat embarrassing, test is performed to rule out the presence of sperm-killing substances in the cervical mucus. The PCT is also used to determine whether you are producing an adequate amount of cervical mucus and whether its consistency is appropriate for the time of your cycle. You and your husband will be instructed to have intercourse after having abstained for two days. Ideally, the test will be performed around mid-cycle, when you are most fertile.

Anywhere from 8 to 24 hours after coitus, you will arrive at the doctor's office, where the physician will remove some mucus from your cervix and examine the sample under a microscope. Ideally, there will be many active sperm present. If the pH level of your mucus is inhospitable to sperm, if there is not an adequate amount of mucus, if the mucus is thick, or if there is an infection or anti-sperm antibodies in your mucus, the doctor will see either no sperm or a large proportion of dead sperm or sperm shaking in place as opposed to moving in a forward direction. The immunobead test, described earlier in this chapter, can be performed to detect anti-sperm antibodies.

A poor post-coital test outcome also can result if your husband's sperm is inadequate or his semen has not reached your cervix. Since your husband's sperm count can vary from day to day and cervical mucus changes throughout your cycle, it's important to repeat the post-coital test two or three times. You may also want to use an ovulation-detection kit to time the PCT to ensure that the test is being done at the right time of the month. If you use a kit, have intercourse the night the kit turns positive and have the PCT performed the next day.

HYSTEROSALPINGOGRAM (HSG)

The HSG is also known as a tubal dye test and can be performed in a hospital outpatient unit or a radiologist's office. The HSG is used to look for blockages in the uterus and fallopian tubes. During the test, dye is injected through the vagina and cervix into the uterus and up the fallopian tubes. No incisions are necessary. As soon as the dye is injected, X-rays are taken to reveal any tubal blockages and show the shape of the uterus as well as any abnormal growths such as fibroids, polyps, or scar tissue. The HSG can also detect congenital abnormalities such as a septum dividing the uterus or a "bicornuate," or double uterus. The test takes about 20 minutes, but it can be painful. Again, you may want to take Motrin or Advil about a half-hour prior to the test.

Like most diagnostic tests, the HSG is not foolproof. If the injection of dye causes a spasm in the fallopian tubes, it may appear as a blockage on the X-ray. On the flip side, an HSG can occasionally be curative if it "blows open" blocked tubes. Risks of the HSG include infection.

HYSTEROSCOPY

Performed in a hospital under local or general anesthesia, a hysteroscopy enables the doctor to directly view the inside of the uterus and opening to the fallopian tubes. The doctor looks through a scope placed through the vagina and cervix into the uterus. During the procedure, the doctor can cut away or laser away polyps, fibroids, and adhesions. Risks include an untoward reaction to anesthesia, perforation of the uterus, and infection.

LAPAROSCOPY

This test is more invasive, since it requires one or more incisions to be made in the abdomen. While you are under general anesthesia in a hospital, the doctor inserts a tube called a laparoscope through your navel and pumps carbon dioxide into your pelvic and abdominal cavity. The gas lifts the abdominal wall away from the organs, giving the doctor a clear view.

During the laparoscopy, the physician will examine the outside of your uterus, fallopian tubes, and ovaries, looking for adhesions, growths, endometriosis, and other abnormalities that may be impairing fertility. In some cases, the doctor may be able to remove adhesions or endometriosis implants during the laparoscopy. After the operation, you may experience temporary pain in your shoulders as the residual carbon dioxide rises before it is absorbed harmlessly by the body. Risks associated with a laparoscopy include an untoward reaction to anesthesia, damage to internal organs, and infection.

Ask the doctor whether she can perform a laparoscopy and endometrial biopsy at the same time. Combining more than one test into a single procedure saves time and money and spares the patient the stress of another operation. It also helps the doctor reach a diagnosis sooner.

PART II
TREATING
INFERTILITY

CHAPTER 5

TREATING INFERTILITY WITH SURGERY AND DRUGS

For some infertility patients, surgery, drugs, or a combination of both is all they need to have a baby. For instance, if you've had a series of early miscarriages, your problem may simply be a lack of progesterone. Taking progesterone supplements during the first trimester could very well do the trick by keeping your uterine lining dense enough to nourish the embryo before a placenta is able to form fully and take over the job. Or if you have fibroid growths inside your uterus and are not ovulating regularly, surgery to remove the fibroids and a drug to regulate ovulation may be all you need, provided your husband's sperm is normal and nothing else is preventing pregnancy.

This chapter will focus on the most common surgical techniques and drug and hormonal therapies being used today to help infertility patients get pregnant and carry their babies to term. Of course, surgery and drug treatment alone may be inadequate or inappropriate in your case. Or your doctor may want to combine surgery and drug therapy with one of the assisted reproductive procedures described in the next chapter.

On average, the cost of surgery runs between $3,000 and $10,000 a couple, depending on what needs to be done. Certain problems, such as mild endometriosis, can be treated at the same time they are diagnosed during laparoscopy. This spares the patient a second operation and holds down medical costs. Other variables affecting costs include a doctor's fee, the hospital's overhead, and what part of the country you live in.

FERTILITY SURGERY TO HELP WOMEN

Fertility surgery on women is usually performed with a technique called "endoscopy." Endoscopy involves inserting a rigid, tube-like instrument (an endoscope) into the pelvic region either through the cervix or through one or more small incisions in the abdomen. The procedure, considered very safe, can be done under general anesthesia, usually on an outpatient basis.

An endoscope is a telescope of sorts, equipped with a lens and a fiber-optic light source. Using an endoscope, the physician can directly examine the inside or outside of the reproductive organs from various angles. Endoscopes also serve as conduits that enable the doctor to insert surgical instruments to repair damage or remove abnormal growths or scar tissue.

When the endoscope is inserted through the vagina and cervix and into the uterus, the procedure is called a hysteroscopy. When incisions in the abdominal wall are used, it is called a laparoscopy. Both hysteroscopy and laparoscopy may be used in the diagnosis phase as well, and laparoscopy is used during GIFT and ZIFT procedures (see Chapter 6).

HYSTEROSCOPY

Therapeutic hysteroscopy is usually ordered if the HSG (the tubal dye test described in Chapter 4) indicates a problem inside the uterus. The most common uterine problem is the presence of polyps or fibroids. These benign growths can be large enough to interfere with a fertilized egg's ability to implant, or they can block the entrance to one or both fallopian tubes.

In addition, scar tissue (adhesions) or a septum (wall of tissue dividing the organ in two) may be found in the uterine cavity. Polyps, fibroids, adhesions, and septums all can contribute to an increased miscarriage rate, and all can be corrected through hysteroscopy.

Adhesions typically occur in women who have had repeated surgical abortions. If the adhesions are moderate to severe, the woman will menstruate infrequently or not at all, or will have a very light menstrual flow. Adhesions can be cut away with scissors or destroyed with electricity.

The rate of restored fertility is very high after surgery, except among women with advanced disease. Most doctors will perform a follow-up hysteroscopy, or hysterogram, to ensure that the uterine cavity is normal before the couple resume attempts to get pregnant.

LAPAROSCOPY

One of the most common uses of laparoscopy is the removal of adhesions that form in the pelvic region outside the uterus. Caused by endometriosis, infection, or previous surgeries, adhesions can block or contort the reproductive organs. During laparoscopy, adhesions are either cut away with scissors, cauterized (burned off) with electricity, or vaporized with a laser beam. There is always a risk that adhesions may return as a result of the laparoscopy itself, however. Be sure to ask your doctor about this risk beforehand.

Another relatively common use of laparoscopy is to destroy endometriosis—the pieces of uterine lining that had abnormally migrated from the uterus and implanted themselves on other pelvic organs, such as the ovaries. The implants can be removed electrosurgically, with laser or heat, or through aspiration (vacuum pressure). The success rate of laparoscopy is higher when the extent of endometriosis is either mild or moderate. Most pregnancies occur within six months of the surgery. Laparoscopy also can be used to remove ovarian cysts.

The most challenging laparoscopic procedure is opening

blocked fallopian tubes. When performed by a skilled and experienced surgeon, tubal laparoscopy can be very successful.

Like hysteroscopy, the success rate of laparoscopy depends on the doctor's judgment and experience as well as the type and severity of the problem being treated. Before you submit to surgery, don't be coy about asking your doctor how many laparoscopies he or she has performed. You also should be given an idea of your chances of success.

FERTILITY SURGERY TO HELP MEN

VARICOCELECTOMY

As explained in Chapter 2, a varicocele is basically a varicose vein that forms above the scrotum in about 8 percent of men. A varicose vein forms when the tiny valves inside a small segment of the blood vessel are faulty, allowing blood to pool. In the case of a varicocele, this pooling is believed to raise the temperature inside the scrotum, creating a less-than-ideal environment for sperm development.

While a varicocele does not always result in infertility, it is diagnosed in 20 to 30 percent of men whose sperm quality is below normal. The doctor will want to rule out other causes of male infertility before recommending a varicocelectomy. The operation, performed through a small incision in the lower abdomen, involves tying off the affected vein segment. This relatively simple surgery can be done on an outpatient basis under local or general anesthesia. It carries few risks and cannot worsen your partner's sperm problem, although there is no guarantee that it will improve the sperm count. It may take three to six months or even longer before any sperm improvement is seen.

About 30 percent of men who undergo varicocelectomy will

have no improvement. Of the 70 percent of patients who do see some improvement, about 30 to 40 percent may ultimately impregnate their fertile wives, compared with 15 to 20 percent of men with an untreated varicocele. Side effects include groin tenderness, which becomes permanent in a minority of cases.

DUCTAL SURGERY

Another common cause of male infertility is a blockage in the microscopic ductal system in the testicles and penis through which sperm travel and mature. Some men are born with these blockages; others develop them as a result of an infection. Because the ducts are so tiny, ductal surgery is most successful when performed with the help of a microscope. Sometimes the damage is too extensive to fix. Even when the operation is successful, the patient may have to wait up to two years before his sperm motility becomes normal. Your husband should ask the surgeon about his experience and success rate with ductal surgery before consenting to the operation.

DRUG THERAPY

There is a variety of safe and effective drugs that can considerably raise your chances of becoming pregnant—and staying pregnant. Since reproduction hinges on a properly functioning endocrine system, most of these so-called "fertility drugs" act on the hormonal system. The most commonly used drugs induce, regulate, or increase ovulation.

OVULATION INDUCTION

If you have irregular periods or do not ovulate, your doctor is likely to prescribe an ovulation-induction drug, such as clomiphene citrate or human menopausal gonadotropin (Pergonal).

Even if you ovulate normally, you may be given one or both of these medications in order to increase the number of eggs you ovulate each month. Ovulating multiple eggs, known as "superovulation," increases the likelihood that at least one of them will meet with sperm and fertilize, either naturally or through artificial insemination. Superovulation is also used to produce multiple eggs that are necessary for in-vitro fertilization.

In addition to inducing ovulation, clomiphene and Pergonal allow your physician to track your menstrual cycle more closely and help you schedule intercourse or artificial insemination on the days you are most fertile. Ovulation drugs also can help correct a timing problem in the second half, or luteal phase, of your menstrual cycle.

Clomiphene citrate, sold under the brand names Clomid and Serophene, should not be prescribed before the patient has undergone a fertility workup. Taken in pill form, clomiphene is the first type of ovulation drug most fertility specialists prescribe. It induces ovulation in 80 percent of patients who fail to ovulate or who ovulate irregularly. The typical dose is one or two pills per day for five days beginning on day 3 to day 5 after your period starts. Ovulation should occur about a week after taking the last pill. It is important to keep an accurate BBT chart while on clomiphene because the drug tends to lengthen the first half of your cycle by a few days (see Chapter 4 for information about the BBT chart).

If you do not conceive, your menses will occur about 14 days after ovulation. If your temperature is elevated for more than 17 days after ovulation, you should take a pregnancy test.

Clomiphene works indirectly by fooling the hypothalamus into believing there is an estrogen deficiency in the body. The hypothalamus signals the pituitary gland to secrete extra FSH and LH, which stimulate the ovaries to produce an egg follicle. In some women, clomiphene therapy results in the production of

more than one egg per cycle. The pregnancy rate with clomiphene is close to that of naturally fertile couples. If there are no
other factors impairing fertility, about 40 percent of couples will
be pregnant after six months of clomiphene therapy and almost
75 percent will be pregnant after a year. If pregnancy occurs as a
result of a clomiphene cycle, there's a 5 percent to 10 percent
chance of having twins. More than two babies are produced in
less than 1 percent of those cases. The miscarriage rate among
women who get pregnant while on clomiphene is the same as in
the fertile population (10 percent to 15 percent).

Clomiphene is also used by men in an effort to increase
sperm count. Since the male reproductive system is not cyclical,
the man must take clomiphene daily for several weeks at a time
and should not expect to see an improvement for at least three
months. Although fewer than 50 percent of men who take
clomiphene will see an improvement, they are not prone to the
side effects suffered by many women who take clomiphene.

Physically, clomiphene may cause cervical mucus to become
sticky and thick instead of thin and stretchy around the time of
ovulation. Sperm are often unable to adequately penetrate thick
mucus. Taking estrogen supplements after clomiphene can often
normalize the mucus. Or sticky mucus can be bypassed through
intrauterine insemination, a form of artificial insemination in
which semen is injected directly into the uterus (see Chapter 6).

The next most frequent adverse effect is hot flushes, which
are reported in about 10 percent of patients. About 5.5 percent
report pelvic or stomach pain; and 2.2 percent suffer nausea or
vomiting. Other adverse effects—blurred vision, headaches, diz-
ziness, bloating, shortness of breath, sensitivity to light, breast
discomfort, headaches, heavy menstrual flow or bleeding between periods, depression, nervousness, restlessness, or trouble
sleeping and fatigue—occur in less than 2 percent of women
who take clomiphene.

Psychologically, the most common complaint by women who take clomiphene is mood swings, which can be quite severe. Report any physical or emotional side effects to your doctor.

Clomiphene's effectiveness can be monitored by the BBT chart, ultrasound scans of the ovaries to watch the egg follicles grow, and blood tests to measure the level of estradiol, a form of estrogen, which increases before ovulation.

If you have a history of liver disease, mental depression, or adverse reactions to the medication, you are probably not a good candidate for clomiphene therapy.

You may, however, be a candidate for human menopausal gonadotropin (hMG), which is sold under the brand name Pergonal. More powerful than clomiphene, Pergonal is designed to induce ovulation in women who fail to ovulate on clomiphene or who have irregular periods. It's also used to induce superovulation, the production of many eggs (6 to 20 or more) in a single cycle. In addition, Pergonal is taken by egg donors, who must produce as many eggs as possible, and by men in an effort to increase sperm production. About 90 percent of women who take Pergonal produce multiple eggs.

Pergonal contains the hormones FSH and LH, which are distilled from the urine of post-menopausal women. FSH and LH directly stimulate the ovaries to produce more eggs.

The drug is a white powder that comes in a small glass container called an ampule. The powder is mixed with a sterile water solution and is injected with a syringe into the hip muscle. Typically, women take one to three ampules of Pergonal each evening for 7 to 12 evenings beginning on day 3 of the menstrual cycle. Since Pergonal should be injected around the same time each day or evening, often when the doctor's office is closed, have your doctor or nurse teach your partner, a family member who lives nearby, or a neighbor how to administer the injection. Some women can learn to inject themselves.

Because everyone responds differently to Pergonal (response rates can even differ from cycle to cycle in the same woman), frequent blood tests are performed to ensure that you are taking the correct dose. These blood tests measure the level of estradiol produced by the egg follicles as they mature. Estradiol testing is usually coupled with ultrasound scans of the ovaries to monitor the growth of the egg follicles.

When the largest follicle is mature (16 millimeters in diameter or larger), injection of another drug, human chorionic gonadotropin (hCG), triggers ovulation within 24 to 48 hours. Estradiol tests and ovarian scans should be done every day or every other day while you are on Pergonal to help the physician monitor your response to the drug, properly schedule an hCG shot, and pinpoint your most fertile time. In addition, hCG is frequently administered during clomiphene cycles.

Frequent scans and blood tests also help avoid Pergonal's most dangerous side effect, "hyperstimulation syndrome." This rare but rather painful enlargement of the ovaries occurs when too many follicles are produced in response to the Pergonal. Hyperstimulation syndrome can be easily avoided with frequent blood tests and ovarian scans. In general, the greater the number of follicles, the greater the risk for hyperstimulation. If your doctor suspects you are at risk for the syndrome, the hCG shot may be withheld.

Hyperstimulation syndrome can vary from mild to severe. In most cases, bed rest at home, with cessation of physical activity, is all that is necessary. Very rarely is hospitalization necessary, since the syndrome will disappear on its own. If pregnancy does not occur, the symptoms will improve 7 to 10 days after the hCG injection. If a patient does conceive, the symptoms will last longer, usually two to three weeks.

Other adverse effects, which occur in 20 percent to 25 percent of women on Pergonal, include swelling at the injection site, bloating, mood swings, and mild abdominal pain.

A recent study led by Alice S. Whittemore, M.D., Ph.D., professor of Epidemiology at Stanford University School of Medicine, indicated that fertility drugs may possibly increase the risk of ovarian cancer, but its findings were far from conclusive. The study, published in November 1992 by the *American Journal of Epidemiology,* found that the risk of ovarian cancer was 1 in 10,000 in the general population, while women who took fertility drugs and conceived had a risk of 3 in 10,000 and those who took fertility drugs but did not conceive had a risk of 27 in 10,000. It is important to note that the type of fertility drugs used by the women studied was unknown, and the number of women included in the study was very small. Furthermore, it was impossible to tell whether the cancers actually were caused by the drugs or by the underlying fertility problem or whether there was a family history of ovarian cancer.

According to the Food and Drug Administration, about 12.5 million prescriptions have been written for Clomid and Pergonal since the drugs hit the market in the 1960s and '70s, respectively, and the FDA has received only six reports of ovarian cancer in the United States possibly associated with fertility drugs. Nonetheless, Merrell Dow U.S.A., the maker of Clomid, and Serono Laboratories, Inc., the maker of Pergonal, now include a warning of ovarian cancer risk on the drugs' labels.

Despite the inconclusiveness of the widely publicized Stanford study, many women who have taken fertility drugs or are contemplating doing so have expressed alarm to their doctors. But, "at present, there is no need to change medical practice regarding use of fertility-enhancing drugs," according to Robert Spirtas, a public health specialist, and colleagues at the National Institutes of Health's Center for Population Research. In a February 1993 commentary in *Fertility and Sterility,* however, Spirtas does suggest that patients receiving fertility drugs be advised "as to the possible increased risk of ovarian cancer" and that physicians take a complete history of all fertility drugs ever taken by their patients "along with a family history of cancer of any kind," as well as the patient's Social Security number, address, and phone number. "Such information," Spirtas and colleagues wrote, "will help physicians contact their patients should more definitive evidence of a causal relationship between fertility drugs and ovarian cancer be found."

About 20 percent of women who conceive during a Pergonal cycle will have multiple pregnancies; about 85 percent of these patients will have twins and 15 percent will have triplets or more. Premature-delivery rates associated with Pergonal are slightly above average, primarily owing to the frequency of multiple fetuses. The miscarriage rate is also higher—20–25 percent—as compared to the normal population's miscarriage rate of 10–15 percent. This higher rate is probably due to earlier recognition of spontaneous abortions, the fact that women on Pergonal tend to be older, and the frequency of multiple fetuses.

Unlike clomiphene, which costs about $4 to $7 a tablet, Pergonal costs about $50 per ampule—that's $350 to $1,800 per cycle, depending on dosage and duration of treatment. As with all drugs used in infertility treatment, check with your health insurer first to learn whether your plan covers these medications. To reduce expenses, ask your doctor if you can use a combined therapy of first clomiphene, then Pergonal, to cut the amount of Pergonal you need to take each cycle.

The pregnancy rate for clomiphene with intrauterine insemination is 10–15 percent per cycle; with clomiphene and Pergonal with IUI, 15 percent; and with Pergonal and IUI, about 15–20 percent.

Women with polycystic ovarian disease and others who have a high level of LH and a low or normal level of FSH may be given a different injectable drug, Metrodin, which is actually follicle-stimulating hormone. Administration, side effects, and multiple births are similar to those of Pergonal. Often, a combination of Pergonal and Metrodin is used.

Women who fail to ovulate can be given a natural hormone known as gonadotropin-releasing hormone (GnRH), sold under the brand names Factrel and Lutrepulse. Lutrepulse can be administered through a portable intravenous pump to simulate a natural cycle. This simulation usually results in the production of a single egg follicle as opposed to the multiple follicles produced by Pergonal. Some women dislike the pump because of its bulk and the fact that they must wear it for two to three weeks each cycle.

In recent years, doctors have begun using synthetic GnRH, known as "GnRH analogs," to increase the effectiveness of Pergonal and Metrodin. These analogs, sold under the brand names of Lupron and Synarel, are taken as injections or nasal sprays. They cause the woman's pituitary gland to gradually stop producing LH and FSH, which are needed to stimulate an egg follicle to grow. In the absence of LH and FSH, the woman's ovulation functions can be completely controlled by Pergonal. This regimen will often increase the number and quality of eggs produced each cycle and will help prevent premature ovulation (releasing the egg into the fallopian tube before the physician has a chance to give you a shot of hCG).

Since GnRH analogs prevent LH secretion, they also can be used in in-vitro fertilization cycles to prevent premature ovulation, allowing the doctor to retrieve the eggs surgically. In egg-donation procedures, GnRH analogs are often used to synchronize the recipient's menstrual cycle with that of her donor. Doctors also administer GnRH to help certain women who suffer from endometriosis. With the menstrual cycle temporarily halted, the endometriosis often recedes. This creates an interlude of several months after GnRH treatment has been stopped during which the patient has a better chance of becoming pregnant.

GnRH side effects may include hot flushes, mood swings, and other symptoms associated with menopause if it is taken alone for several months. Other possible side effects include headaches and nausea. Menopausal-type symptoms are not usually seen when Lupron is given in combination with Pergonal and Metrodin.

In some women, the pituitary gland secretes too much prolactin—the hormone that stimulates the breasts to produce milk. High prolactin levels can be caused by tiny, benign tumors in the pituitary or a hyperactive pituitary, and the condition can be aggravated by birth-control pills, painkillers, or alcohol. Elevated prolactin may also be attributed to kidney, thyroid, or adrenal gland disease. Elevated prolactin levels in non-pregnant women can interfere with ovulation. To correct this problem, the doctor may prescribe bromocriptine, which is sold under the brand name Parlodel. Taken orally once or twice daily, bromocriptine returns prolactin levels to normal in about 90 percent of cases, and about 85 percent of patients will ovulate.

As discussed in Chapter 2, the empty egg follicle must pump out sufficient amounts of another hormone, progesterone, in order to create a healthy endometrium capable of sustaining a fertilized egg. When there is a progesterone deficiency, a fertilized egg may be flushed out during your period before you realize that you conceived. To compensate for a diagnosed or suspected progesterone deficiency, the doctor may prescribe natural progesterone supplements. These supplements come in the form of vaginal suppositories, injections, or capsules. Because the capsule form must be prepared by hand, it is more expensive than the other forms (about $100 for a 10-day supply), and not all pharmacies stock the ingredients. Since the body eliminates excess progesterone, many fertility specialists will prescribe the supplements as a precaution even if there is no direct evidence of a deficiency, especially during IVF and GIFT cycles.

The male hormone testosterone is prescribed for certain men with a low sperm count, but the treatment is controversial. Taken in high doses for 10 weeks, testosterone greatly reduces sperm production in the hope that sperm will "rebound" in much greater numbers after the drug is stopped.

Even if both partners' hormonal systems are working properly, they may be infertile because of a bacterial infection such as chlamydia and mycoplasma. Antibiotics are given to clear up bacterial infections and restore the couple's fertility potential. The most common antibiotic taken by infertile couples is Doxycycline, although other broad-spectrum antibiotics are used. If an infection in one partner is diagnosed, both partners should be treated simultaneously, since bacteria tend to bounce back and forth during intercourse. It's vital that antibiotics be taken in the proper dosage and for the proper amount of time (usually 7 to 10 days). Otherwise, the bacterial infection can come back with a vengeance.

CHAPTER 6

ASSISTED REPRODUCTIVE TECHNOLOGIES

When the average person thinks of infertility treatment, the first thing that springs to mind is in-vitro fertilization. That is not surprising, given all the publicity IVF has received over the years. It explains why so many patients come to a fertility clinic asking for IVF right off the bat, sometimes before a definitive diagnosis has been reached.

In reality, no more than 15 percent of people experiencing fertility problems will resort to IVF or its related technologies, according to a 1988 report from the U.S. Office of Technology Assessment. Artificial insemination, for example, is less expensive and far less invasive than IVF, although its success rate is lower. Nonetheless, artificial insemination has helped countless women become pregnant since 1866, the year the first documented case of artificial insemination was performed in the United States.

This chapter will describe the various forms of artificial insemination as well as the gamut of advanced assisted reproductive technologies (ART) that are becoming more and more routine in fertility clinics across the country. Unfortunately, the more elaborate an ART procedure is, the more costly it becomes. Fortunately, the pregnancy and birth rates associated with these technologies get a little bit better every year as researchers learn more about the subtleties of human reproduction and infertility doctors refine their techniques. Flush with options unimagined a generation ago, infertile couples have never had more reasons to be optimistic.

FERTILE IDEA

The success rates given in this chapter are based on national surveys or on a single clinic that reported results in a reputable medical journal. Use these numbers, along with your physician's success rates, to help you decide which treatment to pursue and when and how long to repeat a treatment before trying something else. But remember that your personal chances of success are based on your age, your unique set of circumstances (biological, psychological, and financial), as well as your ability to adhere to the often rigorous protocols these treatments demand.

ARTIFICIAL INSEMINATION (AI)

One of the oldest approaches to infertility treatment, artificial insemination is used on tens of thousands of women each year who cannot become pregnant through intercourse for a wide array of reasons. Because of its relative simplicity, many couples with unexplained infertility turn to AI before trying any other treatment.

There are varieties of approaches to AI, but they all have at least two things in common: sperm are delivered to the female reproductive tract through a long, thin tube called a catheter; and the treatment is recommended only if your fallopian tubes are open and there are no infections or substantial abnormal growths inside your uterus. In most instances, you will take drugs to enhance and trigger ovulation in order to increase the odds that pregnancy will occur with AI. Basal body charts, LH surge test kits, frequent ultrasound scans of the ovaries, and blood-estradiol tests are used in an effort to time the AI to coincide with ovulation.

AI falls into two major categories: artificial insemination-husband (AIH), which uses your partner's semen; and donor insemination (DI), which uses semen from a donor, usually through a sperm bank.

Provided your tubes and uterus are healthy, your fertility specialist is likely to suggest AIH if your partner has a low sperm count, poor sperm motility, abnormal semen consistency or volume, anti-sperm antibodies, sexual dysfunction, anatomical abnormalities, or retrograde ejaculation. AIH also allows the doctor to bypass any cervical or cervical mucus problems you may have.

DI may be recommended if your partner lacks sperm, has a marked reduction in his sperm count, motility, or both; or has too many deformed sperm in his semen. Genetic defects, sperm allergy, vasectomy, and sexual dysfunction are other indications for DI. Single and lesbian women have turned to DI in order to have children. More about donor sperm and sperm banks is explained later in this chapter.

On average, it takes about six AI attempts before pregnancy occurs, and costs $500 to $1,500 per cycle, depending on which fertility drug or drugs you are taking. If you are using donor sperm, the cost will be a few hundred dollars higher per cycle. You may take a pregnancy test as early as 14 days after the insemination.

AIH or DI is possible with each of the three AI methods in common use today: Cup insemination, intracervical insemination, and intrauterine insemination.

CUP INSEMINATION

This simplest form of AI is typically used when both partners appear to be fertile but the man cannot, for some reason, have normal intercourse. It is also used when the woman needs to take drugs in order to ovulate. During the procedure, semen is injected into the vagina via catheter. A flexible rubber "cup" is then inserted into the vagina to cover the cervix, much as a diaphragm is used. The cup prevents the semen from leaking out, thus allowing more sperm to swim toward the tubes and descending egg. You may resume your normal activities immediately after the procedure. You remove the cup the next day. Cup inseminations are infrequently used because other AI methods are more effective.

INTRACERVICAL INSEMINATION

Intracervical (into the cervix) insemination is recommended when the sperm quality and quantity are moderate to low or if the infertility stems from unknown causes. During intracervical insemination, the vagina is opened with a speculum and semen is injected, through a catheter, into the cervix. After the procedure, you lie quietly on your back for about 10 minutes before resuming your normal activities. According to a small controlled study with donor semen performed by researchers at Oregon Health Sciences University, the monthly pregnancy rate for intracervical insemination was only 5.1 percent, compared with 23 percent for intrauterine insemination.

INTRAUTERINE INSEMINATION (IUI)

Intrauterine insemination is the most costly of the AI methods, but it appears to be the most cost-effective, since sperm are delivered directly into the uterus where they can readily swim up the fallopian tubes. Among the more common reasons to use IUI are: a diagnosis of hostile cervical mucus or anti-sperm antibodies in the mucus, a moderate to low sperm count, or any combination of these problems. IUI also is used when the cause of infertility is unknown.

The reason IUI is more expensive is that the sperm must first be "washed," or spun in a centrifuge. Washing removes prostaglandin, a hormone-like compound that normally is filtered out by cervical mucus. If prostaglandin enters the uterus, severe cramping and infection can occur. Washing also eliminates bacteria, chemicals, and dead and non-motile sperm from semen. Another benefit of washing is that it fosters "sperm capacitation," the process by which the cap at the top of each sperm cell falls away, revealing a pointier head underneath. Capacitation must occur to enable the sperm to penetrate an egg. The minimum number of motile sperm required for IUI is 1 million after it has been washed and prepared for the insemination. With fewer than 1 million motile sperm in the sample, there is almost no chance that pregnancy will occur. At least 1 million motile sperm also are required for procedures such as IVF and ZIFT. Only when micromanipulation is used (see descriptions later in this chapter) are smaller numbers of motile sperm a possibility.

When the husband's sperm is used, he must bring a semen sample to the doctor's office within 60 minutes of producing it. If he lives some distance away, he can ask to produce the sample in a locked examination room in the office. It then takes about an hour to prepare the sperm for insemination. After the prepared sperm is injected into the woman's uterus via catheter, some doctors ask that she lie still for about 10 minutes before resuming her normal activities.

The realities of artificial insemination are such that a husband and wife can conceive their child while they are in separate rooms—or separate counties. If you are bothered by the clinical nature of these procedures, ask your partner to be with you, holding your hand, during the insemination.

SUCCESS RATES OF AI

Success rates are functions of both the timing and the source of the infertility. Men with poor-quality sperm but normal sex drives are less likely to impregnate their wives via AIH than are men with good sperm but low sex drives or impotence. Likewise, women with healthy tubes and no endometriosis or pelvic adhesions have an excellent chance of becoming pregnant with donor sperm if their husband's is inadequate. Also, women under 35 are more likely than older women to get pregnant after an AI.

Overall, the pregnancy rate for AI during a cycle without fertility drugs is about 10 percent, and 10 to 15 percent when Clomid is used prior to AIH. A Clomid/Pergonal cycle coupled with IUI has a 15 percent pregnancy rate, while a Pergonal-only IUI cycle has a 15 to 20 percent pregnancy rate.

Taking the best cases with the worst, the pregnancy rate is about 10 percent to 15 percent per cycle for all forms of AI. By comparison, fertile couples have a 20 percent to 25 percent chance of pregnancy per cycle through intercourse. About 40 percent of women who undergo AIH will be pregnant after six attempts.

The cumulative DI pregnancy rate among women under age 30 is about 74 percent after 12 treatment cycles. That rate slips to 61.5 percent among 31- to 35-year-olds, and 53.6 percent of women over age 35 will be pregnant after 12 DI cycles.

If, after 10 to 12 AI attempts, there is no pregnancy, it's probably time to try a more aggressive treatment.

ADVANCED REPRODUCTIVE TECHNOLOGIES

In-vitro fertilization—"test-tube babies"—is the most well known of the advanced reproductive technologies. IVF is also a catchall term used to describe three other related techniques—

gamete intrafallopian transfer (GIFT); zygote intrafallopian transfer (ZIFT); and tubal embryo (stage) transfer (TE[s]T).

What these procedures have in common is that eggs are physically removed from your ovaries and later transferred back to your body in a fertilized or unfertilized state. In most cases, you first take fertility drugs to induce superovulation. The number of eggs produced during superovulation may reach 20 or more, and can vary from cycle to cycle. The average is about 10. Once the eggs are mature, around mid-cycle, the doctor will do an egg-"harvesting" procedure. The harvesting employs a hollow needle that gently sucks the egg out of its follicle while the patient is under intravenous sedation. The needle reaches the ovary either through the vagina, using an ultrasound picture as a guide, or through the abdominal wall during a laparoscopy.

Donor eggs can be used with any IVF procedure, as can donor sperm. The transfer is carefully timed so the woman's uterus is ready to receive and nurture any embryos that might arrive as a result of medical intervention. Since an average of four eggs or embryos are transferred per cycle, more than one in five IVF procedures—22 percent—result in multiple fetuses. The cost of IVF runs from $3,000 to $8,000 per attempt. If pregnancy does not occur within four to six cycles, most doctors will advise against further treatment with that particular technique.

IN-VITRO FERTILIZATION

IVF is usually recommended when the fallopian tubes are blocked and surgery to clear the blockage is either unsuccessful or not desired. Since fertilization is attempted outside the body for IVF, infertile couples who undergo the procedure can learn whether the husband's sperm are even capable of penetrating his wife's eggs, and whether the wife's eggs are healthy enough to be fertilized.

After the eggs are harvested, they are placed in a petri dish along with sperm in the hope that fertilization will occur. Any fertilized eggs are incubated for two days to allow them to divide into the so-called "pre-embryo" stage. An average of four pre-embryos (if that many fertilized) are then transferred to the uterus in the hope that at least one will implant and grow. Any additional pre-embryos can be frozen for use in future IVF attempts, sparing the woman another harvesting operation. If pregnancy occurs, the extra pre-embryos may be kept frozen for several years should the couple want more children, or they can be donated to another infertile couple. Couples wishing to keep their pre-embryos are charged a monthly maintenance fee up to $50 or $100 a month, depending on the IVF program. At least 75 percent of pre-embryos can be expected to survive the freezing and thawing process.

GAMETE INTRAFALLOPIAN TRANSFER (GIFT)

Considered the most natural form of IVF, GIFT also is proving to be the most successful. Common diagnoses among GIFT candidates include unknown causes and mild endometriosis. For GIFT to work, at least one of the woman's tubes must be clear and the uterus free of major abnormalities. Her partner's semen analysis should be normal. There is, however, no way of knowing at the time of a GIFT procedure whether the woman's eggs are capable of being fertilized. Therefore, many doctors are placing any extra harvested eggs in a petri dish and mixing them with sperm to see whether they fertilize. If fertilization occurs, they can have the pre-embryos frozen for a future IVF attempt.

During GIFT, gametes (the medical term for sperm and egg cells) are mixed in a special catheter and injected into one or both fallopian tubes, where it is hoped they will fertilize in the environment that nature intended. The best eggs are identified by a specialist called an embryologist. GIFT is performed via laparoscopy, which requires general anesthesia.

TUBAL EMBRYO (STAGE) TRANSFER

TE(s)T is identical to IVF in every way except that the pre-embryos are transferred to the fallopian tubes instead of the uterus 48 hours after fertilization in a petri dish. Any perceived advantages of TE(s)T over IVF were thrown into doubt, however, by a study published in *Fertility and Sterility* in February 1992. Jose P. Balmaceda, M.D., and colleagues at the University of California looked at 42 patients who used donor eggs that were fertilized to the pre-embryo stage outside the body. Twenty-two patients had the pre-embryos transferred to their uterus and 20 had them transferred to their fallopian tubes. The pregnancy rates were almost identical for both groups—54.5 percent after uterine transfers and 57.9 percent after tubal transfers. The researchers concluded that the quality of both the embryo and the uterine lining appeared to be "significantly more important than the time of entrance of an embryo to the uterine cavity in determining its chances of implantation."

ZYGOTE INTRAFALLOPIAN TRANSFER

Like IVF, ZIFT enables the doctor to ascertain whether the sperm indeed penetrated the egg. ZIFT also allows subsequent cell divisions to take place in the fallopian tube. In ZIFT, harvested eggs are placed with sperm in a petri dish and allowed to fertilize to the zygote stage, a process that takes about 24 hours. A zygote is the name given to the cell that is created after fertilization but before the first cell division. The embryologist will select the best zygotes, usually up to four, to be transferred to the fallopian tubes. ZIFT is sometimes referred to as pronuclear stage transfer (PROST).

FERTILE IDEA

Before deciding whether to attempt any ART procedure, ask your physician under what circumstances would the cycle be canceled. A transfer of gametes or embryos, or even the egg-harvesting procedure itself, is canceled in about 10 percent of cycles, usually because of poor response to fertility drugs. Other reasons for cancellation: if the woman's ovary releases the eggs spontaneously before the doctor has an opportunity to retrieve them surgically; if she fails to produce enough eggs to make the attempt worthwhile; or if retrieved eggs fail to fertilize outside the body during an IVF, a ZIFT, or a TE(s)T cycle.

SUCCESS RATES

With doctors becoming more experienced in assisted reproductive technologies, it is not surprising that the success rates are inching up every year. A 1990 survey of 180 IVF clinics in the United States found live delivery rates of 14 percent for IVF, 22 percent for GIFT, and 16 percent for ZIFT. The latest available data—1991 statistics—from 215 ART programs nationwide found the live delivery rate had increased to 15.2 percent for IVF, 26.6 percent for GIFT, and 19.7 percent for ZIFT. These data were collected by the Society for Assisted Reproductive Technology and the American Fertility Society and published in *Fertility and Sterility.*

"We encourage patients to ask the clinic how many deliveries (live births) they had per egg retrieval," says Mary Martin, M.D., director of the IVF program at the University of California and 1993 president of the Society for Assisted Reproductive Technology. "The difficulty comes if one program talks about pregnancies per [egg or embryo] transfer and another talks about live deliveries," Dr. Martin says. If the programs stick to the same kind of reporting standards, patients will be better able to compare success rates before selecting a clinic, she explains. In addition to considering the clinic's overall birth rates, patients also should take their particular form of infertility into consideration. "If a couple has a severe male factor problem, they will know their chances [of conceiving] are zero, so the [clinic's success] rate won't apply to them," Dr. Martin says.

AGE CONSIDERATIONS

Women over age 30 who are considering IVF "should avoid unnecessary delay before they start treatment," investigator Seang Lin Tan and colleagues recommend in the June 6, 1992, issue of the *Lancet*. Their conclusion stemmed from a study of more than 2,700 women who underwent IVF in the United Kingdom. The study found that 54 percent of the women under age 34 were pregnant after five IVF treatment cycles, with 45 percent carrying to term. Their pregnancy and birth rates approach those reported in the population at large. However, in women aged 35 to 39, only 39 percent were pregnant at the end of five IVF cycles and 29 percent gave birth. Among women aged 40 and older, just 20 percent conceived after five IVF cycles and 14 percent gave birth.

U.S. statistics for 1990 also showed that pregnancy and live birth rates drop dramatically after age 39. The pregnancy and live birth rates for women over 40 undergoing IVF was 11 percent and 7 percent, respectively, compared with 19 percent and 15 percent for women ages 35 to 39. Women over age 40 undergoing GIFT had a 17 percent pregnancy rate and 9 percent live birth rate compared with a 27 percent pregnancy rate and 21 percent live birth rate for women ages 35 to 39.

FERTILE IDEA

The reason pregnancy and birth rates are low at many IVF centers is that IVF is usually sought by older women in the first place. When you are looking for an IVF clinic, ask for referrals from Resolve, the American Fertility Society, or friends who have obtained fertility treatment. Ask the clinic what its clinical pregnancy and live birth rates are overall and for women your age. If the IVF clinic you are evaluating has a lower-than-average success rate, ask how old the average woman is when she is accepted into the program and how old she is when she conceives with IVF. Since many couples take a two- or three-month break between IVF cycles, it is not unusual for the woman to be 34 when treatment is initiated and 36, 37, or even older by the time treatment is discontinued.

DONATION

DONOR SPERM

Each year in the United States, an estimated 10,000 babies are born as a result of donor insemination. Donor sperm used in conjunction with IVF and its related procedures account for several thousand more births annually.

Donor sperm is most commonly used when the husband's sperm count or motility is extremely low or he is sterile. Sperm donation also is indicated if the husband has non-correctable ejaculatory dysfunction or a genetic disorder such as Huntington's disease, hemophilia, or chromosomal abnormalities that pose a high risk to any child he fathers.

Using fresh donor semen used to be the norm. When it was discovered that AIDS can be sexually transmitted, fresh donor semen fell out of favor. Today, only frozen donor semen is used, even though pregnancy rates using frozen semen are lower than those using fresh semen. "A complete sexual history should be obtained to exclude as donors individuals who might be at high risk for HIV and/or who have multiple sexual partners," state sperm bank guidelines issued by the American Fertility Society.

After the donor produces a semen sample, the sample is frozen in liquid nitrogen (a process called cryopreservation) and quarantined for six months. The donor undergoes an AIDS test at the beginning and end of the quarantine period, since it can take up to six months after exposure to the AIDS virus for antibodies to be detectable through a blood test. Only when the donor's AIDS tests are negative will his sample be released to an infertile couple. Sperm has been safely cryopreserved for up to 10 years.

The American Fertility Society's guidelines regarding AIDS testing were developed in accordance with positions adopted by the FDA and the Federal Centers for Disease Control. Be sure to ask whether the sperm bank your doctor uses strictly adheres to those guidelines.

The guidelines further recommend that prospective donors have a complete physical exam prior to donation and follow-up exams afterward. Doctors conducting these exams should look for discharge from the urethra, genital warts, and genital ulcers, as well as other abnormalities that suggest infection. Men with a family history of genetic defects or hereditary diseases such as cystic fibrosis or hemophilia must be rejected.

Despite careful screening, recipients should be aware that there is "no absolute method of completely ensuring that infectious agents will not be transmitted" through donor insemination, the guidelines point out. "But following the guidelines, in addition to adequate history-taking and exclusion of individuals at high risk for HIV (e.g., homosexuals, bisexuals and intravenous drug users), should make that possibility remote."

In the past, sperm donors were primarily college students, graduate or medical students. Today, they come from all walks of life. Once the men are deemed healthy and free of known genetic diseases, only those with exemplary sperm are accepted as donors. Confidentiality of both the donor and the recipient is guaranteed at most sperm banks, although the guidelines encourage sperm banks to maintain permanent confidential records of donors, including their genetic workup, and to make the anonymous record available on request to the recipient and any resulting offspring.

Thanks to express mail service and the ability to transport frozen sperm in insulated bottles, you can use a sperm bank in another state. The sperm bank or your doctor can give you a list of potential donors, identified by number. Additional information on each donor generally includes blood type (including Rh factor), race, religious/ethnic background, hair and eye color, height, weight, build, years of schooling, vocation, and hobbies. Many couples choose a donor whose physical attributes are similar to the husband's.

Sperm donors are paid roughly $30 for each semen sample accepted by the sperm bank. When a donor's sperm has impregnated 10 women, the sperm is no longer sold, to lower the possibility that half-siblings will unwittingly marry. Cost of donor sperm to the recipient ranges from about $300 to $500 per sample, depending on the sperm bank. You and your husband will be asked to sign a statement assuming full custody and responsibility for any child produced with donor sperm and acknowledging that the risk of birth defects or other problems are the same as if you were conceiving on your own.

FERTILE IDEA

Many men with impaired fertility view the use of donor sperm as a threat to their virility, and experience a host of negative emotions stemming from the fact that any child conceived with donor sperm will not share the infertile parent's genetic heritage. If your partner is reluctant to use donor sperm, he may wonder whether his sperm can be mixed with the donor's prior to the insemination. However, many specialists believe mixing diminishes the quality of the donor sperm. It's a better idea to make love with your husband the evening after the donor insemination. The idea that his sperm might fertilize your egg after all may alleviate your partner's anxiety to some extent.

Another option is choosing a known donor such as your husband's brother. The advantage is that you can pass on some genes from your husband's family. If the donor is a friend, you'd know firsthand that he is healthy and has no genetic diseases in his family. Sperm from a known donor should be quarantined for 180 days while the donor undergoes the same evaluation and screening (including AIDS testing) that anonymous donors must go through under the fertility society's guidelines. Bear in mind that using a known donor can pose moral, ethical, and even legal problems down the line, as well as emotional problems should the child find out who his biological father is. If you choose not to tell your child the details of his or her conception, you may feel more comfortable using an anonymous donor, which ensures that your privacy will be protected.

DONOR EGGS

The hottest new trend on the fertility circuit is egg, or "oocyte," donation. Since 1986, some 67 U.S. fertility clinics began offering egg donation, and, according to a survey by the

American Fertility Society, those clinics reported 547 donor-egg transfers in 1991 alone. As of March 1992, the survey found, an estimated 900 donor-egg transfer cycles had taken place in the United States, resulting in about 275 pregnancies. Reports of live births were unavailable.

Most candidates for donor eggs, according to the American Fertility Society, are women with premature ovarian failure that is uncorrectable by drug therapy. Other candidates include women whose ovaries have been surgically removed or destroyed by chemotherapy or radiation therapy, and women who have had persistently poor egg or embryo quality during previous attempts at IVF or other ART procedures. Women who have no eggs or poor-quality eggs but whose reproductive organs are healthy "become pregnant more often and are more likely to reach term with the use of donor [eggs]," states the fertility society guidelines for egg donation.

For several reasons, egg donation is far more complicated, and thus far more expensive, than sperm donation. The egg donor must take fertility drugs and undergo surgery to remove her eggs. For her efforts, she is generally paid $500 to $2,000 by the infertile couple, who also pick up the tab for the donor's drug regimen and egg-retrieval surgery. Egg recipients are also charged for recruitment and screening of potential donors. Even if the donor is known, the guidelines recommend that she should undergo medical and genetic screening aimed at protecting the recipient from infections, such as AIDS, and the baby from hereditary problems. The guidelines also say that couples entering an egg-donor program should be offered a choice of assuming "the low risk of acquiring HIV by using fresh embryos" or having the embryos frozen and quarantined so the donor can be retested for the AIDS virus six months later. The quarantine option, of course, raises the overall price of the procedure and decreases the success rate.

Other expenses the recipient must cover are the drugs she is likely to take prior to the donor-egg transfer. The drug therapy is designed to synchronize her menstrual cycle with the donor's and to prepare the lining of the recipient's uterus to accept implantation. Cycle synchronization is necessary because eggs cannot be frozen with current technology.

Donated eggs can be used with IVF, GIFT, ZIFT, or TE(s)T. If the husband's semen analysis is normal, his sperm will be used to fertilize the donated eggs. If his semen analysis is abnormal or he is at high risk for passing a hereditary disease to his offspring, donor semen can be used. The ART technique used helps determine the costs to the infertile couple—costs that range from $2,500 to more than $15,000 per cycle, with no guarantee for success. National surveys reveal that the pregnancy rate for IVF using donor eggs is 35 percent to 40 percent each cycle.

The majority of women who seek donor eggs are between ages 35 and 55, according to the American Fertility Society survey. "In our experience . . . these individuals enjoy pregnancy success rates similar to those of younger women," the survey authors wrote in the July 1992 issue of *Fertility and Sterility*. Furthermore, they wrote, women who use donor eggs "do not appear to place themselves at undue obstetrical risk."

Nonetheless, egg-donor guidelines issued by the society recommend that potential recipients over age 40 undergo a thorough evaluation, including psychological assessment and cardiovascular screening, and be told of any potential health risks before being approved to receive donated eggs.

FERTILE IDEA

When you are looking for an egg-donor program, experience is the key. The fertility society survey found that the more donor-egg cycles a facility had completed, the higher its pregnancy rate. Programs that had performed more than 100 donor-egg cycles reported a 35 percent pregnancy rate per egg transfer, compared with a 16 percent pregnancy rate among those that had performed fewer than 10 donor-egg transfers. You should also make sure that the program follows the American Fertility Society's guidelines.

According to the fertility society, the majority of IVF programs require you to identify your own egg donor, although an increasing number of fertility clinics are beginning to recruit their own pools of anonymous donors. Anonymous egg donors are usually college students or young mothers who don't want any more children. Like sperm donors, most egg donors are acting on an altruistic streak, although many admit the money is also an incentive.

If you will be selecting from a donor pool, be sure the clinic tests and screens out women with a family history of genetic problems. The clinic also should conduct a psychological evaluation of potential donors and accept only those who are emotionally balanced and seem unlikely to back out of the program or try to pursue custody of a child who is conceived with their egg.

Most egg-donor programs require that the anonymous egg donor remain anonymous. In fact, donors generally are not told whether a pregnancy has occurred. If you choose a known donor, such as a sister or a friend, you'll need to resolve many emotional issues for both you and your donor prior to undergoing the procedure. Meeting with an infertility counselor first can be helpful.

DONOR EMBRYOS

When the husband and the wife both have severe problems with their gametes, they may turn to donor embryos. The embryos usually come from an infertile couple who became pregnant with IVF and had their leftover pre-embryos cryopreserved. If they do not plan a subsequent pregnancy or do not wish to pay a monthly maintenance fee for the freezing tank, they may donate their extra pre-embryos to help another infertile couple. Some fertility clinics in need of donor pre-embryos will discount their fee to couples in exchange for their extra pre-embryos. Cost to the recipient ranges from $500 to $2,000, depending on how long the pre-embryos have been frozen. The live birth rate for a frozen embryo transfer cycle ranges from 7 percent to 15 percent, depending on the experience of the clinic.

SHOULD YOU TELL?

If you and your husband opt to use donor gametes or embryos, you must decide whether to disclose this fact to friends, family, and, eventually, to any child born as a result of donor technology. You must weigh the pros and cons of telling and figure out what you feel most comfortable doing. It's often helpful to discuss these issues with an infertility counselor so that you are sure you have considered all the ramifications of your decision.

Despite the growing popularity of gamete and embryo donation, little research has been done on its emotional implications. One study showed that couples who told friends or relatives that they used donor sperm to conceive wound up regretting the disclosure. Their regrets stemmed from the potential emotional trauma to their child should the child learn about his or her origin through the grapevine.

MICROMANIPULATION

Some of the newest techniques in the world of ART—
manipulating eggs and sperm under a microscope—are aimed at
couples who have the most difficulty getting pregnant. The
groups of patients who qualify for micromanipulation include
husbands whose live sperm counts are very, very low; wives who
have abnormal eggs; and patients who have had poor fertilization results during previous IVF procedures.

PARTIAL ZONA DRILLING (PZD)

Partial zona drilling helps couples conceive when the husband's sperm is found to be incapable of penetrating the zona,
or egg's shell, on its own because of poor motility or low sperm
concentration.

In PZD, eggs are surgically removed from the wife or a
donor, and a specially trained surgeon uses microsurgical tools
to drill a hole partially through the egg's shell. The husband's
sperm is then introduced in hopes that a single sperm cell will
have an easier time making its way to the egg's nucleus. If the
egg fertilizes, it is transferred to the wife's womb.

In most cases, the people who opt for this costly technique
are turned off by the idea of using donor sperm. Partial zona
drilling should not be considered until a couple has tried IVF or
one of its related procedures at least twice but failed to achieve
fertilization or had a low fertilization rate; or if the husband's
sperm count is so low that it does not meet the minimum re-
quirement for IVF. PZD appears to be most successful when
there is a significant male-factor problem as opposed to problems with the woman's eggs. Other techniques that are similar to
PZD include Suzi (Subzonal Insertion of Sperm) or ICI (Intracy-
toplasmic Injection of sperm) directly into the nucleus. ICI has
been shown to be the most successful; however, very few centers

in the United States offer the option at this time.

Cost of PZD can hit $10,000 or more per attempt. Of PZD procedures performed on 163 patients at the Cornell center during an 18-month study, 39 (24 percent) resulted in pregnancies, and 35 (about 22 percent) of those pregnancies resulted in a live birth.

ASSISTED HATCHING

With assisted hatching, an egg is fertilized in a laboratory and allowed to divide to the embryo stage (24 to 48 hours after fertilization). The embryo's outer core is then punctured microscopically before being transferred to the uterus. This process has been shown to increase the implantation rate. Since assisted hatching is so new, it is only offered at a few select fertility centers. Be sure to find out if the fertility center you are working with does micromanipulation procedures such as PZD and Hatching, and Suzi.

SURROGACY

As we learned from the infamous Baby M case, having another woman give birth to your child packs potentially explosive legal and ethical dilemmas. Infertile couples who choose this route should do so only after considerable thought and investigation into the laws overseeing surrogate parenting, which vary from state to state. In many states, surrogacy is simply illegal. Couples wishing to hire a surrogate should be prepared to pay at least $10,000 to the surrogate and another $10,000 to a lawyer. The couple may also have to pay for the surrogate's obstetrical care and hospital expenses.

There are several reasons couples consider surrogacy: the wife lacks a uterus or has a disease that would be aggravated or life-threatening during pregnancy; the surrogate mother can carry a baby conceived from the adoptive parents' egg and sperm, from her own egg fertilized with the adoptive father's sperm, or from her own egg fertilized with a donor's sperm. Any of the reproductive technologies may be used, but artificial insemination is the most common. Some infertile couples use a relative or friend to serve as a surrogate. Attorneys who specialize in surrogacy and adoption can also help infertile couples find a surrogate.

CHAPTER 7

COPING EMOTIONALLY AND FINANCIALLY

For most couples, infertility is a heartbreaking, emotionally devastating life crisis that threatens to shatter their self-worth along with their dreams of parenthood and their bank account. By communicating well, resisting the temptation to blame your partner or yourself, learning everything you can about your condition, and wringing the most out of your insurance policy, you and your partner can weather this storm, for the majority of infertile couples wind up with a baby (or babies) in their arms.

COPING EMOTIONALLY

The yearning for children of your own can encompass a spectrum of strong, sometimes overwhelming emotions: desire, longing, hope, love, hate, jealousy, envy, betrayal, hostility, sadness, resentment, rejection, hopelessness, anxiety, despair, depression, confusion, desperation. According to psychological researchers, anxiety and depression seem to be the predominant emotions among couples undergoing infertility treatment.

If you've already endured a few treatment cycles, you are probably familiar with the pattern. Couples often describe it as a roller-coaster ride of high hopes and anxiety followed by crushing depression with each failed attempt at conception. "I cry every time I get my period," says Donna, the mother of a 5-year-old boy who tried for a second child for three years before giving up.

The intensity of emotions changes over time. For some couples, the emotions get more intense as pregnancy seems to become more and more elusive. Others learn to reduce their expectations as they come to realize that they may be in treatment for the long haul. This lowering of expectations can be helpful even as you fortify your resolve to do everything possible to have a baby.

Because the "roller coaster" is inherent in infertility treatment, there is no way to get off the ride completely, points out Diane Clapp, R.N., medical information director at Resolve, the Somerville, Massachusetts-based infertility advocacy and support organization. "It's important to be an informed consumer, to be aware of your chances of success given your age and diagnosis. However, even in the bleakest of circumstances, there always is that flicker of hope which propels people to the top of that roller coaster."

As infertility drags on, Clapp says, couples learn to protect themselves from hope. It's not quite pessimism that they are experiencing, but more a denial of hope. "I've known a lot of people who wish they didn't have hope. Then it would be easier for them to go through it," says Clapp, who endured many years of infertility before adopting and subsequently becoming pregnant.

One key to maintaining your sanity through the infertility ordeal is to view each treatment cycle *not* as a potential answer to your prayers, but as a *single step* toward your ultimate goal. In artificial insemination, for instance, your statistical probability of getting pregnant rises with each attempt. Helping matters is the fact that you and your doctor can fine-tune the protocol with each AI cycle, such as adjusting drug dosages and fiddling with the timing of the insemination. Remember that scientists learn more from their mistakes than their successes.

The intensity of your emotions also change as you try different or more advanced treatments. One study found that the level of anxiety among women undergoing egg retrieval (a minor surgical procedure) for an IVF was similar to the anxiety experienced by women about to undergo major gynecological surgery. Patients who enter an IVF program tend not to be depressed, however. "This is perhaps not surprising given that depression is generally associated with loss, and couples embarking upon treatment are still hopeful about having a child," writes Susan Golombok, of the Clinical and Health Psychology Research Center in London, who reviewed the research on the psychological effects of infertility for a 1992 article published in *Human Reproduction.*

Golombok points out that how patients cope with their infertility seems to influence whether they will suffer psychological problems. People who isolate themselves or use alcohol to try to reduce tension "had higher levels of emotional distress than those who engaged in . . . strategies such as seeking information about their treatment or making a plan of action," she writes. Paying attention to the latest findings in infertility research and devising a treatment plan, she suggests, can make you feel more in control.

Reading an informative book on infertility, joining a support group, finding a good doctor, and knowing what questions to ask are other ways infertile couples can wrest some control over their fate. Says Clapp: "Become an advocate for yourself."

Mustering the emotional strength to become a self-advocate is not always easy, particularly when you are awash with negative feelings and your self-esteem is in the basement. If you are undergoing treatment already, take action during the time in your cycle when you feel strongest and most hopeful—a few days before and after an insemination or egg transfer. Then, if you get your period two weeks later, you can read the material you have gathered or the action plan you have written.

How can you tell whether your emotional upheaval is normal for your circumstances? Golombok's article points to a profile set forth by one group of researchers of an infertile woman most likely to have emotional difficulties: a young woman who endorses a religion that places an emphasis on child-rearing, who lacks a confiding relationship with her partner, who is undergoing other life stresses, and who has not been given a diagnosis for her infertility. If you fit this profile, or otherwise feel your negative emotions or impulses are preventing you from deriving any enjoyment from life, it's wise to seek out psychological counseling now. Counseling should come from a psychologist or social worker who has personally experienced infertility or who has counseled other infertile couples. Try as they may to help, some counselors who have never encountered a client with infertility before can do more harm than good.

Infertile women who are clinically depressed, psychotic, or extremely agitated may need a psychiatrist's help. Those experiencing negative emotions normally associated with infertility could benefit from behavioral therapy, anxiety-reduction techniques, and relaxation training. Behavior therapists use a variety of techniques to help patients change their abnormal behavior patterns instead of attempting to analyze the root causes of their problems.

One study of about 50 women in the Behavioral Medicine Program for Infertility, at New England Deaconess Hospital in Boston, suggested that behavioral therapy can make infertility treatment much more bearable. The women attended 10 weekly group counseling sessions, including a 7-hour session held on a Sunday. Husbands attended the first session and the Sunday session.

During each session, participants were shown how to relax their bodies and their minds. They were given stress-management tips and nutritional education and they learned how to do gentle stretching exercises. They also were taught how to transform their negative thoughts into positive ones. Participants were paired up with a "buddy," and buddies were asked to speak with each other at least once a week. All participants were instructed to practice the skills they learned for 20 minutes a day between sessions. The groups were co-led by a behavioral therapist and a "peer counselor"—a woman with infertility who had mastered the behavioral techniques.

Before and after completing the program, participants filled out questionnaires designed to assess their moods. In virtually every case, participants' level of tension/anxiety, depression/dejection, anger/hostility, fatigue, and confusion all declined significantly after therapy.

KEEPING YOUR MARRIAGE ON TRACK

A common fear among infertile couples is that their dilemma will somehow damage or even destroy their marriage. While this certainly has happened in some cases, the fact that you and your husband have begun treatment probably reduces the chance that infertility will spur a divorce.

Two studies in the late 1980s that explored marital and sexual problems among infertile couples found no evidence that they were having major difficulties in these areas. "It seems likely," Golombok writes, "that in order to survive the investigative procedures and reach the stage of embarking upon treatment, the couples need to have a stable marriage and a good sexual relationship; thus, only those with a good marriage and who do not have marked sexual problems ever reach this stage." Of course, if you feel your marriage is in trouble already, you may wish to postpone or suspend infertility treatment in order to get some marital counseling.

One of the major reasons marriages break up is poor communication. Spouses cannot begin to meet one another's emotional needs if they have no clue as to what those needs are. It is particularly important to communicate your feelings effectively while undergoing the stress of infertility treatment. If you feel you are less than a woman if you cannot conceive without medical intervention, share these thoughts with your partner. Thus, he'll realize you need an extra dose of affection and reassurance that you are still feminine and attractive to him. Conversely, if your husband's low sperm count has battered his self-esteem, encourage him to express those anxieties, and give him the reassurance he needs to remember that he is still as appealing as ever to you.

Supporting your husband emotionally right now is extremely important because the chances are you're the only person he may be able to confide in. Research has shown that men tend to keep their personal problems to themselves while women tend to disclose their feelings to close friends and relatives, thus generating a support network. "Women must realize that men respond differently to the crisis of infertility than women do," observes Clapp. "A wife may think her husband doesn't understand if he doesn't express his feelings or throws himself into his work, while in fact he's grieving just as hard as she is. It's just different."

Experts agree it's vital that couples attack infertility as a shared battle to be waged together. Resenting your husband for having a low sperm count when it is beyond his control does nobody any good. Some of the strongest bonds in the human experience occur among soldiers who fight a common enemy side by side. Likewise, you and your husband can solidify your marital bond by forging a united front against your common enemy: infertility—regardless of the source. And if you finally do get pregnant, you will share a unique brand of joy. "As happy as fertile couples are when they get pregnant," one woman who conceived after her ninth AI says with conviction, "we're happier."

COPING WITH FRIENDS AND FAMILY

Couples who openly and diplomatically explain their infertility to their close friends and family members tend to have an easier time coping. This is especially so if you can find someone who has firsthand experience with infertility to talk with. Clapp recommends sharing not only certain facts about your situation, but at the same time telling your confidante what you need—such as a sympathetic ear, or baby-sitting while you go for a treatment. Otherwise, Clapp says, you may be setting yourself up for a barrage of advice that you don't want or need.

Since infertility treatment can disrupt your work schedule, it's also helpful to tell an understanding supervisor what you are going through. Sympathy can work wonders in getting you the time you need off from work for frequent doctor's visits and tests.

But don't expect everyone to be empathetic, or even sympathetic, to your plight. People who don't want children may have trouble understanding your desperation to become parents. People who get pregnant easily may say that there are far greater tragedies in life than infertility. However, Golombok writes, a study in the Netherlands found that more than 40 percent of women and 20 percent of men attending an infertility clinic reported that involuntary childlessness "was the worst thing that ever happened to them."

And then there are the advice-givers. Some people, when they hear you're having trouble getting or staying pregnant, can't help recommending a week in the Caribbean or telling you to "relax." And it seems that everyone knows someone who got pregnant as soon as they stopped trying or the moment after they signed adoption papers. Unless the advice-givers are infertility specialists, chances are their personal prescription for pregnancy is based on one of the myths covered in Chapter 1.

If well-meaning but meaningless advice irritates you, try conveying your feelings to the advice-givers. Tell them you appreciate their concern, but you are under a doctor's care and are doing everything possible to get pregnant. The same goes for family members who try to pressure you to have children. Flatly tell them you have a fertility problem and you're under treatment. Then change the subject.

It's not unusual for infertile women to feel uncomfortable around pregnant women and other people's babies. Presumably, your friends and family members will be sensitive enough to understand when you politely decline an invitation to events such as a baby shower or a baby's birthday party. "You have to sort of protect yourself from painful experiences," recommends Clapp. "I encourage people to give themselves permission to send a gift certificate or check instead of attending the shower."

But be flexible. Your tolerance for baby-oriented activities might change over time. One woman undergoing infertility treatment said the first baby shower she attended was the hardest emotionally. After that, baby-centered events became easier.

When you discuss your infertility with friends and family, don't feel compelled to tell them all the gory details, says Clapp. "Controlling who knows and how much people know, and telling them what you want from them by way of support are real important first steps to controlling your social life."

As odd as it may seem, keeping a sense of humor can also help you maintain a sense of control. One husband who routinely ejaculated into a cup for his wife's artificial inseminations said this about sperm washing: "I understand that my semen has to be washed, but how do they get the sperm onto those tiny little hangers afterward?"

COPING FINANCIALLY

Like most areas of medicine today, infertility treatment doesn't come cheap. AI can cost $1,000 or more a month, including fertility drugs and tests. IVF fees range from about $3,000 to $8,000 or more per cycle. Many couples who abandon treatment do so because they run out of funds. It is not unusual for couples to borrow or take on an extra job to have enough money to pursue their pregnancy dream. And there is little argument that the wealthy and gainfully employed are more likely to have access to infertility treatment than Americans of lesser means.

Those fortunate enough to have a good health-insurance policy may find that at least some of their medical expenses are covered. According to a study published in 1991 by Marian Damewood, M.D., director of the In-Vitro Fertilization Program at the Johns Hopkins Hospital in Baltimore, the majority of insurance carriers cover between 50 percent and 80 percent of "conventional" infertility treatments—that is AIs, surgeries, and drug therapies; the majority of American health insurers do not cover IVF and related technologies. Ironically, insurers often reimburse for surgery to correct blocked fallopian tubes, even though the chances of conceiving after tubal surgery are lower than they are for conceiving through IVF with no tubal surgery.

If both you and your husband are members of group health plans provided by your respective employers, you're in an enviable situation. Whatever bills or portion of bills your insurance policy doesn't cover can be submitted to your husband's insurer for reimbursement.

Getting familiar with your health-insurance policy and your husband's should be step No. 1 before launching into infertility treatment. If your employer offers a choice of more than one type of health plan (such as Blue Cross-Blue Shield and a health-maintenance organization), ask your personnel department or benefits counselor about each plan's coverage for infertility before making a decision. Companies that self-insure should also be queried. You may be surprised to learn that your insurer covers AI and IVF, albeit on a limited basis. Or perhaps the policy covers drugs or surgery to treat endometriosis or will reimburse you for a diagnostic laparoscopy. Your drug plan may even cover the extremely expensive ovulation drug, Pergonal.

As of January 1993, at least nine states—Maryland, Rhode Island, Hawaii, Texas, Arkansas, Connecticut, Massachusetts, New York, and California—had passed laws mandating health insurers to provide coverage of infertility treatment, including assisted reproductive technologies, according to the American Fertility Society and Damewood's study. The scope of coverage in those states varies, and proposed legislation in other states to mandate infertility treatment coverage moves at a glacial pace.

One of the arguments used to persuade lawmakers to vote in

favor of these bills is that infertile people's insurance premiums are used to pay for fertile people's maternity services, so a portion of fertile couples' premiums should be used to help infertile couples. Moreover, Damewood argues, covering infertility treatment is economical in that it can save the insurer the expense of tubal surgeries. If your claim for reimbursement is rejected, try using these arguments in your appeal. You can also use them with employers that self-insure in order to get at least some of your expenses covered.

The way doctors bill also can influence whether you get reimbursed. For instance, a bill for "endometriosis treatment" would be covered because it is a disease in and of itself. Billing for "infertility treatment" may not be covered, even if the diagnosis was endometriosis as a cause of infertility. While your policy may not cover ART, it probably covers ultrasound scans, blood tests, hormonal therapy, and other treatments you may be receiving. Ask your doctor whether he or she is willing to bill you for these components individually.

The power of suggestion is another tool at your disposal. Carol's insurer covered three AIs and three IVF procedures. After the first three AIs failed, her doctor suggested she try at least three more before advancing to IVF. The doctor put his recommendation in writing to Carol's insurance company, and she enclosed her own letter explaining that it was cheaper to cover three more AIs than a single IVF. She also mentioned that her chances of being pregnant after three more AI cycles were at least equal to, if not greater than, her chances of getting pregnant after a single IVF. In closing, Carol mentioned that the owner of her company pays a high price to insure his people well. A few weeks later, Carol received a letter back from her insurer, who agreed to fund three more AIs. To her delight, Carol became pregnant before having to resort to IVF.

FERTILE IDEA

If you have no insurance coverage or inadequate coverage, you may want to consider taking on a part-time job or borrowing the money to subsidize your treatment. If you have office skills, offer to volunteer your services to help your doctor's office staff in exchange for free treatment. One patient took that approach one step further. A free-lance writer, she worked out a barter deal with her doctor under which she created advertisements for his brother's gourmet food store in exchange for free medical care, including sperm washings, ovary scans, and artificial inseminations. The only thing she paid for were laboratory fees for blood tests. If you've already spent your last dime on treatment, and your doctor feels you still have a good shot at success, he or she may be willing to give you a month or two of free treatment.

BRAVE NEW WORLD

The patchwork quilt that is the American health-insurance system is likely to fall by the wayside if President Clinton makes good on his campaign promise to reform the way health-care providers are reimbursed. The new system will be a boon or a bust for infertility patients, depending on whether their needs are covered. Regardless of the nature of any universal health-care plan that is put into place, chances are there will always be private insurance carriers ready to pick up the slack. Employers may offer supplemental insurance plans as a benefit to lure good employees, and individuals will always be free to purchase additional coverage on their own.

WHEN TO QUIT

Each time you try and fail at one of the assisted reproductive technologies, you are faced with the question of whether to keep trying or to give up. Some couples decide on their limits before they begin treatment. Others feel they're doing themselves a disservice unless they try every technology available. Still others let their finances dictate how much they are willing to endure.

"It's a good idea to have at least two medical opinions" of your prognosis before deciding whether to quit, says Clapp. "You may not choose to try all the options, but at least you will know what they are."

You should also consider your quality of life and how much it has been disrupted so far by infertility treatment. Would continuing treatment or trying a more invasive procedure further erode your quality of life?

If you feel stuck at a crossroads, or you and your husband disagree on what to do next, consider taking a two- or three-month breather from treatment. Use this time to work out your differences, save some money, and regain the strength you need to push on, if that is what you choose to do.

If you decide enough is enough, you may still want to keep your options open should a new technology become available down the road. In the meantime, begin the adoption process.

The process of letting go of your dream of having children can take many months or even years, so be patient with yourself. And remember that human beings are innately adaptable, and you will eventually come to terms with your infertility and actually be comfortable with the hand you were dealt. If you continue to have difficulties coping, reach out to professionals or support groups for help.

CHAPTER 8

Like stories of childbirth you hope to share with your friends someday, stories about infertility are unique to each couple. Even if you and the woman sitting beside you in the waiting room have an identical medical problem, you differ in regard to your emotional response to infertility, your relationship with your husband, your choice of treatment, and your financial wherewithal to pursue advanced reproductive technology if it becomes necessary.

Here are stories of three women, how they discovered their infertility and how they coped with it. The stories are based in part on composite sketches, with certain names and details— including those of the women and their doctors—altered to protect their privacy.

ZOË AND ALEX, A COUPLE IN THEIR MID-30S

Zoë freely admits it: "I had a career, but I never wanted to be a career woman. I wanted to stay home with my kids."

So when she married her second husband, Alex, in December of 1985, they began their quest for a family immediately. To their delight, Zoë was pregnant two months later. But a week after rejoicing in her positive pregnancy test, Zoë began to bleed. She thought it was an early miscarriage, but the bleeding continued for two weeks before she went to her gynecologist.

Tests quickly revealed that Zoë was experiencing an ectopic pregnancy. She underwent emergency surgery, which left her with only one fallopian tube. She realized that this halved her fertility potential, but she didn't give it much thought. She and her husband resumed their efforts to get pregnant.

Zoë tracked her ovulation cycle with temperature charts and ovulation-predictor kits. She appeared to be producing eggs, and her husband's sperm were healthy (he had a son from a previous marriage). Yet after 18 months, Zoë was still trying to get pregnant.

The gynecologist she had been going to since 1975 was "conservative" and did not live up to the title of "infertility specialist" he had printed on his business cards. "I really liked Dr. Marconi, but our feeling was that if you can't do anything else, then say you can't do anything else. It was actually my husband who finally confronted him and said, 'Look, is there anything else that can be done?' The doctor said, 'Well, we could check to see if the remaining tube is open.' "

The couple asked for a referral to a specialist who could give them more options. The doctor said he would get back to them. He never did.

Almost a year later, Zoë read a book about infertility which motivated her to go to Pennsylvania Hospital's Philadelphia Fertility Institute.

Emotionally Zoë thought she was holding up just fine—until she went to Pennsylvania Hospital for her initial meeting with a member of the staff. "The woman said something about being interviewed—and well, I just started to cry," Zoë recalls. "My husband answered all the questions. I couldn't even talk."

The interviewer, Ellen, had seen this cascade of sadness and despair before in other patients. "I think you really need help to get through this, because if you get accepted into our program, and it doesn't work, I don't know what's going to happen to you," she said, handing Zoë the telephone number of an infertility counselor.

The interview process was followed by a battery of medical tests to assess Zoë's hormonal balance, the patency of her remaining tube, and the health of her uterus and cervical mucus. The worst of the tests, Zoë recalls, was the endometrial biopsy. "I went for the biopsy alone. It wasn't supposed to be a big deal, but I almost broke the nurse's hand. This pain was ridiculous."

After the biopsy, Zoë regrouped and drove 45 minutes back to her husband's physical-therapy office, where she worked as office manager. After work, she went to her sister-in-law's house and burst into tears. "The whole thing is so traumatic when you can't have a baby or you think you can't have a baby," Zoë says. "It's an awful emotional roller coaster."

Within a couple of months, all the tests on Zoë were complete. By then, she was 35 and deemed an ideal candidate for the institute's in-vitro fertilization program because of her age, and adhesions in her abdominal cavity stemming from the tubal pregnancy. She was told that the success rate was less than 20 percent and that the average patient undergoes three IVFs before she gets pregnant or gives up.

To Zoë, whose alternative was the loss of a life-style she had always envisioned for herself, the potential of having an IVF baby was well worth the emotional risks. Alex was more pragmatic. "If it doesn't work, we can spend our time traveling and enjoying each other," he told his wife.

Fortunately, Zoë's insurance policy covered virtually all of the costs for up to five IVFs. Although only $100 came out of pocket, the expense of the treatment really hit Zoë when she purchased her first doses of Pergonal. "I was writing out a check for seven hundred and ninety-five dollars at the drugstore. I couldn't believe it," she says, wondering what she would have done if she hadn't been insured.

Zoë's regimen of Pergonal shots required her to report to the IVF clinic each afternoon for 12 to 14 days for blood tests and ovary scans. Each morning, she'd call the clinic to learn how much Pergonal to take that day. Each day around the same time, she'd have to track down her husband to give her the shot.

When the time was right, doctors extracted 11 eggs from her ovaries during a virtually painless procedure. The eggs were placed in a petri dish where they were mixed with Alex's sperm. Four of the eggs fertilized and were transferred into Zoë's uterus.

Then came the waiting game. After the egg transfer, Zoë walked with the grace of a ballerina and avoided heavy lifting. She even drove slower. When she returned to the clinic two weeks later, her pregnancy test was positive. News that her hCG level was lower than it should be, however, went in one ear and out the other.

"I was thrilled to death and even got sick to my stomach right away," Zoë recalls. Zoë let her fantasies of motherhood run wild.

But at work the next day, she began to bleed. Her counselor had warned her that the IVF probably would not work the first time. Nonetheless, Zoë was very upset. She told Alex, "I'll never go through this again," even though her counselors, doctors, and nurses all urged her not to give up.

But she was too traumatized. And the trauma and tension had begun to affect her marriage. Zoë grew increasingly jealous of Alex's relationship with his son Seth, who spent every other weekend with them. She vented her jealously and anger over not having her own child by lashing out at her husband. Alex couldn't understand why Zoë couldn't love Seth, too. She did love the boy, but she couldn't get past the fact that the boy would never be hers.

To make matters worse, Zoë's younger sister, already the mother of 8- and 6-year-old boys, decided to try for a girl. "She got pregnant just like that," Zoë said, snapping her fingers. It happened just as Zoë was suffering through the failed IVF. "When my sister got pregnant, that made my life miserable," Zoë recalls.

The sister thought that naming Zoë godmother would help ease her pain. But it had the opposite effect. Zoë was so sick to her stomach and had such a bad migraine the morning of the christening that she asked her sister-in-law to stand in for her. "Now I know why I got sick," Zoë says. "It was all psychological."

Six months later, Zoë changed her mind and decided to try IVF again. "I guess I needed that time to grieve because every time a woman loses a child, whether you're pregnant for a day or three months, you still have lost a child. Even though I was pregnant for only twenty-four hours, in my mind, I was already a mother. I had it all planned out," she explains.

Before the second IVF, Zoë took both Clomid and Pergonal to stimulate her ovaries to produce multiple eggs.

Each time she returned to the clinic for daily monitoring, she saw the same group of women who were also undergoing IVF. In the waiting room, they traded stories and advice and became the best support group Zoë could hope for. Several lived so far from the clinic that they were staying in a hotel near the hospital during the course of their treatment.

"My story was nothing compared to what these girls were telling me. One woman was there for her fifth time," Zoë remembers. "These women made me realize more than anything that it's not going to work the first time, but you can't give up if you really want to have a baby."

Just as in her first IVF, 11 eggs were retrieved and four fertilized and were transferred to Zoë's uterus. Just like the first time, her pregnancy test was positive two weeks later. But this time, the hCG level was up where it should be in a normal pregnancy, and it continued to rise. Two euphoric weeks later, though, Zoë began to bleed again and rushed back to the clinic. An ultrasound revealed that two fertilized eggs had implanted, but one was aborting naturally. The other was right where it should be. Zoë was delighted. "I wanted kids, but I wasn't ready for twins," she says. Jason, a healthy 7-pounder, was born nine months later.

Zoë had no intention of trying IVF for a second child, but miraculously she became pregnant naturally when Jason was nine months old. She took baby Lynn and Jason to a reunion of the first 200 IVF babies born through Pennsylvania Hospital's program. There she learned she was only one of two women in the program who had gotten pregnant spontaneously after giving birth to an IVF baby.

Looking back, Zoë realizes that she never would have found the courage to try IVF a second time if not for the counseling sessions. "I always thought and continue to think of myself as a very strong person emotionally," Zoë says. "Getting counseling to deal with infertility doesn't mean you're weak; it means you're experiencing a normal reaction to an abnormal situation."

YVONNE AND JOSEPH, A COUPLE IN THEIR EARLY 40S

Yvonne and Joseph married when they were in their mid-20s and both fresh out of law school. The two attorneys decided to delay starting a family for at least seven years while they built their respective law practices. Building those practices proved more time-consuming than they anticipated. When their seventh wedding anniversary rolled around, they decided to put off having children for another three years.

"We figured it wouldn't make much of a difference when we had our kids, as long as we had them," Yvonne says. "Anyway, the longer we waited, the stronger our practices became and the higher our income. We wanted to be able to send our children to the best private schools money could buy."

When Yvonne was 35 and Joseph was 36, they abandoned birth control and let nature take its course. Unfortunately, nature had something else in store for them. After one year of carefully timed lovemaking, Yvonne became pregnant, only to miscarry at four weeks. Her second miscarriage occurred six months later, at six weeks' gestation. Saddened by the miscarriages but buoyed by the knowledge that she was capable of becoming pregnant, Yvonne sought help from her gynecologist, who had some experience treating infertility.

A semen analysis showed Joseph's sperm was normal. A laparoscopy revealed that Yvonne had mild endometriosis. The extent of the disease was not enough to impede conception, however, her doctor said, noting that she had gotten pregnant twice already. Temperature charts and ovulation-predictor kits indicated Yvonne was ovulating regularly. Both of her tubes were found to be open, her uterus was healthy, and there were no hormonal balances to contend with.

"I can't see any reason why you have been unable to maintain a pregnancy," her doctor said. "The only diagnosis I can come up with is unknown causes."

To Yvonne, "unknown causes" was more frustrating than finding a problem. "At least if we could pinpoint what was wrong—a blocked tube or something—then we could do something definitive," Yvonne says. "But not knowing is like being in limbo."

Yvonne and Joseph continued trying to get pregnant on their own for another eight months. Then her doctor prescribed the ovulation drug Clomid, coupled with intrauterine insemination. Yvonne and Joseph followed the regimen for six months, to no avail. The next step was combining Clomid and Pergonal followed by IUI. The couple went on with the new protocol for the next three months, but Yvonne's period continued to come like clockwork. They took a two-month break before resuming treatment, this time with Pergonal followed by IUI. Another four months went by with no pregnancy.

By now, Yvonne was 38 and her nerves were frazzled. As her biological clock ticked louder and louder, her desire to become pregnant became more like an obsession. Fears of never having children would spill over into other aspects of her life, including her work. When a client asked her to file a medical malpractice lawsuit because the woman's doctor had failed to diagnose an ectopic pregnancy, Yvonne referred her to another lawyer.

"The idea of suing a doctor for rendering a client infertile hit too close to home," Yvonne explains. "Even though our situations were completely different, my strong emotional reaction to her dilemma made it impossible for me see the situation from the doctor's point of view. Without the ability to anticipate the other side's arguments, I could not prepare an effective case against him."

On a more personal front, both Yvonne and Joseph were faced with parents who badgered them about starting a family. Joseph's mother thought their problem stemmed from too much work-related stress and advised Yvonne to quit her job. Friends recommended that they take a long vacation.

"I couldn't convince anyone that we were doing everything

possible to have a baby," Yvonne recalls. "Even though we didn't know what was wrong, we knew full well that quitting my job or taking a vacation wouldn't cure it."

Finally, Yvonne's doctor admitted he could do no more to help them. He gave her a copy of her medical chart and referred her to a nearby IVF clinic. At first, Yvonne recoiled at the idea of more medical intervention. But Joseph convinced her that it was their only choice.

Dr. O'Toole, director of the clinic, suggested a GIFT procedure coupled with IVF. Any eggs that fertilized in vitro would be frozen for implantation later should the GIFT fail, O'Toole told Yvonne. Hearing that the success rate for GIFT was relatively high compared with IVF, Yvonne's hope was renewed.

She took high doses of Pergonal and was closely monitored to ensure that the drug did not cause her ovaries to enlarge. Yvonne and Joseph had intercourse every 48 hours or so to keep his sperm output at an optimal level. Through frequent ultrasound scans, Dr. O'Toole was able to watch 15 egg follicles mature—seven in one ovary and eight in the other. When the follicles were ripe, he performed an egg-retrieval operation.

During another operation, four eggs and Joseph's semen were placed into Yvonne's fallopian tubes. An embryologist determined that 10 of the remaining eggs were large enough for an IVF attempt. However, 24 hours after those eggs were allowed to mingle with Joseph's sperm, not one had fertilized.

"This was our first clue that perhaps the real problem was with fertilization," Yvonne says, describing her reaction at the time as "shocked." Not surprisingly, the GIFT did not work, either.

Still determined to have a baby, Yvonne and Joseph decided to take another two months off to regroup emotionally. When they returned to the clinic, O'Toole recommended doing a straight IVF with as many eggs as Yvonne could safely produce in a single cycle. This time, 18 eggs were retrieved and all were mixed with Joseph's sperm in a petri dish.

"I remember thinking that this approach just has to work," Yvonne says. "I guess I was in denial. I would not accept the fact that something was wrong with my eggs."

Normally, 75 percent of eggs fertilize with IVF. In Yvonne's case, only two of those 18 eggs fertilized. Yvonne was devastated. She cried uncontrollably as Dr. O'Toole put the two fertilized eggs into her uterus. She had never felt more pessimistic in her life.

In a support group run by the clinic, Yvonne could only cry. She had been through more torment and failures than anyone else in the room. Every conversation with her doctor left her in tears, as well. Joseph, meanwhile, was burnt out by the whole fertility fiasco. He wouldn't attend the support group meetings with his wife. He even toyed with the idea of asking Yvonne for a divorce—not because she couldn't bear his children, but because she had become chronically depressed and bitter. She was nothing like the energetic, positive woman he had married. He feared that Yvonne might turn self-destructive if he left her. So he stayed.

When Yvonne got her period two weeks after the IVF, she simply felt numb. There were no more tears left, it seemed. Dr. O'Toole said their only hope was using a donor egg.

"You mean put some fertile woman's egg in my uterus?" Yvonne asked, horrified.

"Yes," Dr. O'Toole said. "You would pay her a fee of around twelve hundred dollars, and she would take Pergonal and give to you any eggs that she produced. Since all your reproductive organs are working, there's a fairly good chance that you would become pregnant and carry a baby to term. You might even end up with twins."

By now, Yvonne had only contempt for any woman lucky

enough to be fertile. She could not fathom carrying in her womb what amounted to a stranger's child. Joseph encouraged her to give donor eggs a try, but he could not convince her to change her mind.

"I wanted *our* child, not *a* child," Yvonne laments. "Using donor eggs is not acceptable to me. I'd rather adopt. At least this way, neither of us would be more closely related to our son or daughter." For almost a year, Yvonne and Joseph mourned their inability to produce a child they could biologically call their own.

When Yvonne was 40, she called an old law school friend who specializes in private adoptions. Two years later, Yvonne and Joseph became the proud parents of an adopted baby girl.

KATHY AND BRIAN, A COUPLE IN THEIR LATE 20S

So intent were Kathy and Brian on becoming parents that they abandoned birth control one month before their wedding day. "Even if I get pregnant, I'll still be able to fit into my wedding dress," Kathy reasoned.

When Kathy was not pregnant six months later, she began complaining to her gynecologist. "Just relax and have intercourse every other day," the doctor said. Six disappointing months later, the doctor repeated his advice and handed her a set of basal body temperature charts.

Because her husband came from a large family and none of his siblings had ever had a fertility problem, Kathy assumed the problem was with her. She took her temperature and filled in her BBT chart religiously, noting the days she had intercourse and days she was sick or took medication. Kathy also purchased an ovulation-detection kit and arranged lovemaking dates with her husband by telephone so he'd know his responsibility after the workday was over. She watched the telltale rise in her temperature during the second half of her cycle, but her heart would fall each time the temperature dipped a degree, indicating her period was about to begin.

Despite her regular ovulation and menstrual cycles, Kathy, a public-relations consultant, was still convinced there was something in her reproductive tract preventing her egg from reaching her husband's sperm. She begged her gynecologist to do some tests. He first ordered a semen analysis for Brian, a flight instructor. The analysis, performed by a local acute-care hospital, indicated his sperm count was "low to moderate," but, the doctor concluded, certainly sufficient to impregnate his wife. Kathy then underwent an HSG and a laparoscopy. No endometriosis, blockages, or abnormal growths were detected.

"Then why aren't I pregnant yet?" Kathy, increasingly agitated and impatient, asked her doctor. "I don't know," the doctor replied. "You should just relax."

That was the last straw. Kathy asked for copies of all her records and took them to another gynecologist, Dr. Drake, who had been specializing in infertility for more than 15 years. She learned about his practice through a co-worker who had benefited from his expertise several years before.

The first thing Dr. Drake did was a complete medical workup on Kathy, including a vaginal culture and a battery of blood tests. One of those tests turned up a culprit: Kathy and, probably, Brian were infected with a bacteria called mycoplasma. Mycoplasma, Dr. Drake explained, can often prevent conception, but it is easily cleared up with antibiotics. Kathy was elated—and angry that her first doctor missed the diagnosis completely. Noting that Brian's sperm count was less than ideal, Dr. Drake suggested he see a urologist and undergo several more semen analyses.

After finishing their antibiotic prescriptions, Kathy and Brian had intercourse. Kathy arrived at Dr. Drake's office for a post-coital test 12 hours later. The result of the PCT was not at all what Kathy expected. There was not a sperm to be found in her cervical mucus. She left Dr. Drake's office in tears.

A few days later, Dr. Drake suggested the couple begin intra-uterine insemination. IUI, he explained, would circumvent any hostile mucus problems that Kathy might have while giving Brian's sperm a shorter distance to travel to meet her egg. Dr. Drake put Kathy on Clomid so that he could more closely control her ovulatory process. "This IUI has to do the trick," Kathy said to herself. "It's practically delivering sperm on a silver platter."

But one afternoon, two weeks after the IUI, Kathy began to spot blood. Panic-stricken, she phoned Dr. Drake's office. A nurse told her that spotting is not unusual in early pregnancy and not to give up hope. At 2 A.M., however, Kathy was awakened by menstrual cramps. It was at this point that her emotions nearly went haywire. She cried hysterically, punching her pillow, screaming, "What's wrong with me? Why am I being punished? Why can't I be normal and have a baby?"

Brian was more than alarmed. He thought Kathy was having a nervous breakdown, and he didn't know what to do. So he just held her as tight as he could as she cried for three solid hours. It took both of them several days to recover from the episode. Dr. Drake told Kathy that very rarely do these inseminations work on the first attempt. He encouraged her to try again.

In the meantime, Brian received a startling diagnosis from his urologist. He had a varicocele, but it was relatively minor. Since Brian's next two semen analyses basically mirrored his first, the couple continued undergoing IUIs over the next six months. Dr. Drake told them he'd seen pregnancies with worse semen than Brian's.

After three months, Dr. Drake put Kathy on Pergonal so she'd produce more than one egg per cycle and theoretically improve her chances of conception. The side effects of the fertility drugs were minimal, and their health-insurance plans covered about 50 percent of the cost of the drugs, ultrasound scans, blood testing, and IUIs—a total of about $1,500 per cycle. Financially, at least, Kathy considered herself fairly lucky. Not so when it came to practically everything else in her life.

"It felt as though I was being punished by God for doing something terrible, but I couldn't figure out what I had done," she explains. "All around me women got pregnant as easily as drinking a glass of water. I live in a large city, and I see pregnant teenagers all the time. And here we were: mature, stable marriage, good jobs, money in the bank, and no pregnancy. It just wasn't fair."

"But life isn't fair," Brian would tell Kathy during her frequent bouts with depression. However, he too was feeling slighted by fate, particularly when he realized that his sperm count might be the source of their troubles. Brian worked hard to keep his own emotions at bay, reasoning that Kathy was too emotionally fragile to support him. He felt he had to be constantly strong because his wife was so weak.

Kathy, meanwhile, couldn't understand why Brian didn't seem as devastated as she was. His undying emotional strength kept her in an emotionally needy state. One night, though, Brian could keep his feelings in no more. He broke down in Kathy's arms, and she was finally able to tap into her strength in order to support her husband.

After their third failed intrauterine insemination, one of Brian's sisters became pregnant and the other one gave birth. Around the same time, Kathy's best friend conceived on her first attempt. Several of Kathy's co-workers were pregnant; others were forever talking about the trials of parenthood. It seemed that every television commercial Kathy saw was for baby food or diapers. Shopping malls began to look like giant day-care centers. Even a jog in the park was an ordeal; seeing a pregnant women with toddlers in tow would haunt her for days. And she nearly lost her mind whenever she read a newspaper article about teenage pregnancy, crack babies abandoned in hospitals, or a newborn being thrown into a dumpster.

The only way Kathy could think of to cope was to cut herself off not only from her pregnant friends and family members but from everyone with a child under 2. Increasingly desperate to have a baby of her own, Kathy was growing to hate the little creatures.

She and her best friend grew estranged. Her parents and in-laws worried that she would never attend another family get-together. Brian tried his best to be stoic and maintain ties with their relatives, but he felt torn apart inside.

After the seventh failed IUI, Brian decided to see a urologist who specialized in male infertility to confirm his varicocele diagnosis. The urologist, Dr. Norseman, ordered yet another semen analysis, but this one was performed in a highly specialized laboratory. As it turned out, Brian's sperm count wasn't low to moderate, it was downright poor. Only 12 percent of his sperm were motile, and a mere 15 percent were of normal shape. His chance of making Kathy pregnant was minute, regardless of how much Pergonal she took. Correcting the varicocele may or may not normalize Brian's sperm count, Dr. Norseman told him. And even if it did, it would take at least six months after the surgery before they would know for sure.

After what she'd been through and considering how isolated Kathy felt, she couldn't imagine waiting so long for an iffy chance of getting pregnant with her husband's sperm. "I want you to begin thinking about using donor sperm," Kathy told

Brian one night. The idea disgusted him. But he promised to think about it.

Kathy brought up the idea during a session of a Resolve support group they had joined. Brian said he was afraid he might not be able to love a child conceived with donor sperm as much as he could love his own biological child. A psychologist, Yakov Epstein, Ph.D., who was a guest speaker that night had this response: "If the only thing my father contributed to me was his genes, and he wasn't there to help raise me, nurture me, teach me about the world, and give me a set of values, I would not be the same man I am today." Brian thought about those words for many days afterward.

He also thought about Kathy's point that the decision to try donor sperm would be his alone, since she had already made up her mind. Moreover, she argued, if their child was conceived with donor sperm, Brian would be the only father that child would ever know. Brian also thought about Dr. Drake's promise to mix Brian's sperm with the donor's, leaving open the possibility that the child might be genetically his, after all. After much agonizing, Brian said yes. But he wanted no part in selecting the donor.

Kathy was thrilled with his decision, even though she wished he would help her choose. At the same time, Kathy remained fairly pessimistic that an IUI using donor sperm would work. Fearing a reprise of her near-breakdown that followed the first failed IUI, Kathy had been keeping her hopes and expectations at bay.

From a list of some 70 potential donors, Kathy chose one who matched Brian's physical appearance and shared some of his interests.

A week after the donor insemination, Kathy's best friend, Pat, gave birth to a healthy boy. "I have a son, and you're still my best friend," Pat told Kathy, phoning her from her hospital room. "I understand completely if you can't come visit us, but I really miss you."

Kathy decided that her friendship with Pat was too precious to jeopardize. With her heart thumping in her throat, Kathy made the 90-minute drive to see Pat a few days later. As soon as she arrived, Pat put her tiny baby, Scotty, in Kathy's arms. "My God," Kathy said, "how can I hate such a fragile, innocent little thing?" As she held and rocked Scotty, Kathy decided that she could no longer live in a shell, that she must learn to accept her circumstances as one of life's many inequities.

That month, Kathy's period was three days late. But she was afraid to take a home-pregnancy test. She had seen too many of them turn up negative. Anyway, her cycle had been slightly elongated since she began taking fertility drugs.

The next day when her period still didn't come, she called Dr. Drake's office. "You must come in for a pregnancy test," the nurse insisted.

"But I'm afraid," Kathy responded. "Can't I wait until I'm a week late? At least then I'd be fairly certain the test would be positive. I don't know how I'd cope with more disappointment."

"Look," the nurse said, "it's very important to our ability to help you that you take the test now. Even if you're not pregnant, there might have been some fertilization, and a blood test can give us valuable information."

Kathy called Brian at work and asked him to meet her at the doctor's office. "I can't go through this alone, regardless of the outcome," she told him.

Brian arrived just as the nurse finished drawing Kathy's blood. It would be about five minutes before they would know. Kathy and Brian stepped outside to get some fresh air and sunshine while they waited. "I've never been so nervous," Kathy told her husband. "Listen," said Brian, "if the test is negative, we're no worse off than we were last month. We can try donor again, or we can always try IVF. There's still hope."

When they walked back into the office, the nurse was standing in the lab doorway smiling broadly and nodding her head. She showed them the little "+" on the white plastic pregnancy test indicator. Next to the "+" was a small dot, which, the nurse explained, means she performed the test correctly. "You're pregnant," she said. Kathy hugged the nurse, then she hugged Brian, and all three of them cried.

Nine months later, Kathy gave birth to a beautiful baby girl. Within a few weeks, Brian's lingering anxiety over what they did to conceive their daughter dissipated and he loves her as though she were his flesh and blood. On the rare occasion that Kathy thinks about the donor, she feels nothing but gratitude.

APPENDIX

RESOURCES

ORGANIZATIONS

American Fertility Society
2140 11th Avenue South
Suite 200
Birmingham, Alabama 35205-2800
(205) 978-5000

Provides names and addresses of infertility specialists and IVF centers, and booklets on various aspects of infertility.

Resolve, Inc.
1310 Broadway
Somerville, Massachusetts 02144-1731
HelpLine: (617) 623-0744

Non-profit organization supported by membership dues and contributions. Sponsors local support groups; issues newsletters and fact sheets, physician referrals in the United States and Canada, adoption information; lobbies for insurance coverage.

American Self-Help Clearinghouse
St. Clares-Riverside Medical Center
Denville, New Jersey 07834
(201) 625-7101; TDD (201) 625-9053

Provides telephone numbers for statewide Self-Help Clearinghouses, each of which may include local infertility support groups; also provides information on how to launch your own support group.

FURTHER READING

And Hannah Wept: Infertility, Adoption, and the Jewish Couple, by Michael Gold. (Jewish Publication Society, Philadelphia: $19.95.)

Facts for Consumers: Infertility Services. (Office of Consumer/ Business Education, Bureau of Consumer Protection, Federal Trade Commission, Washington, D.C. 20580; (202) 326-3650: 50 cents.) Booklet tells how to interpret success rates and procedures used by IVF clinics.

Getting Pregnant: What Couples Need to Know Right Now, by Niels H. Lauersen, M.D., Ph.D., and Colette Bouchez. (Fawcett Columbine, New York: $12.)

Getting Pregnant When You Thought You Couldn't: The Interactive Guide That Helps You Up the Odds, by Helane Rosenberg, Ph.D., and Yakov Epstein, Ph.D. (Warner Books, New York: $12.99.) Focuses mainly on psychological issues.

Having Your Baby by Donor Insemination: A Complete Resource Guide, by Elizabeth Noble. (Houghton Mifflin Co., Boston: $12.95.)

How Can I Help? A Handbook for Practical Suggestions for Family or Friends of Couples Going Through Infertility, by Diane Clapp, B.S.N., R.N. (Fertility Counseling Associates, Lexington, Mass.: $6.)

How to Get Pregnant with the New Technology, by Sherman J. Silber, M.D. (Warner Books, New York: $14.99.)

Living with Endometriosis, by Kate Weinstein. (Addison-Wesley Publishers, Reading, Mass.: $10.95.)

Preventing Miscarriage: The Good News, by Jonathan Scher, M.D., and Carol Dix. (Harper Perennial, New York: $10.)

What You Can Do About Infertility, by Pamela Patrick Novotny. (Dell, New York: $3.99.)

GLOSSARY

Adhesions: Scar tissue in or around the pelvic organs that may or may not interfere with fertility.

Anovulation: Complete lack of ovulation; no eggs released during a woman's menstrual cycle.

Antiphospholipid antibodies: A type of protein that attacks blood-clotting components and may trigger a miscarriage.

Anti-sperm antibody: A type of protein that attacks sperm.

Artificial insemination (AI): A technique in which a doctor injects semen, either from the husband (AIH) or a donor (DI), directly into a woman's cervix or uterus during her most fertile time of the month.

Assisted reproductive technology (ART): A term used to describe in-vitro fertilization and other interventions infertility specialists use to help egg meet sperm.

Azoospermia: Absence of sperm in semen.

Basal body temperature (BBT): The body's core temperature at rest.

Basal body temperature chart: A grid used to track basal body temperature, which normally rise and falls at different intervals during a woman's menstrual cycle.

Bilateral oophorectomy: Surgical removal of both ovaries.

Bromocriptine: A medication prescribed for non-pregnant women with a hormonal imbalance that causes them to produce breast milk.

Cauterize: To destroy tissue by burning.

Cervix: The neck of the uterus that connects to the vaginal canal.

Cervical mucus: The mucus in the cervix that normally grows copious and stretchy around time of ovulation to help sperm along the journey to the egg. It also serves to filter out many non-sperm components of semen.

Corpus luteum: The empty follicle, or sac, left behind in the ovary after ovulation that then produces estrogen and progesterone.

Cryopreservation: Preservation of semen or pre-embryos by freezing them in liquid nitrogen.

Diethylstilbestrol (DES): A drug prescribed for pregnant women in the 1950s and '60s to prevent miscarriage. DES was banned after it was found to cause reproductive defects in many children exposed to the drug in the womb.

Dry cervix: Lack of sufficient mucus in the cervix caused by a hormonal imbalance, an injury, or surgery.

Egg follicle: The fluid-filled sac in the ovary in which an egg ripens.

Egg-retrieval surgery: A surgical technique in which eggs are suctioned out of the ovaries in preparation for IVF, GIFT, or a related procedure.

Embryologist: A specialist who concentrates on the fertilization and growth of embryos.

Endocrine system: The glands and tissues that secrete hormones into the bloodstream.

Endometrial biopsy: Examination of a small sample of uterine lining under a microscope to compare its age with the day of the cycle the woman was in when the sample was taken.

Endometriosis: A disease in which the lining of the uterus migrates to other regions of the body, usually in the pelvic region.

Endometrium: The inner lining of the uterus that grows each month and is flushed out during the menstrual period or remains intact if conception has taken place.

Endoscopy: Examination of internal organs with a tube-like instrument equipped with lenses and a light source.

Epididymis: A long, coiled tube in the scrotum that carries sperm to the vas deferens.

Estrogen: A group of female hormones vital for sexual development and reproduction; secreted primarily by the ovaries but also by the adrenal glands and, during pregnancy, by the placenta.

Fallopian tubes: The ducts through which eggs travel from the ovaries into the uterus.

Fibroid: A non-cancerous tumor found in the wall of the uterus.

Follicle-stimulating hormone (FSH): A hormone produced by the pituitary gland that stimulates egg maturation in the ovaries.

Fructose test: A test for a type of sugar that normally is present in semen.

Gamete: Medical term used to describe both eggs and sperm.

Gamete intrafallopian transfer (GIFT): An ART procedure in which eggs and sperm are injected into the fallopian tubes.

Gonadotropin-releasing hormone (GnRH): A reproductive hormone secreted by the hypothalamus. GnRH stimulates the pituitary to secrete FSH and LH.

Human chorionic gonadotropin (hCG): A hormone that is produced by the placenta during early pregnancy; hCG stimulates the ovaries to produce other hormones—estrogen and progesterone—which are needed to maintain the pregnancy.

Hyperstimulation syndrome: A temporary condition that results when the ovaries become extremely enlarged, causing significant abdominal swelling and discomfort.

Hypothalamus: A small region of the brain that coordinates the function of the nervous and endocrine systems.

Hysterosalpingogram (HSG): An X-ray that allows the physician to view the size and shape of the inside of the uterus and fallopian tubes; also known as the tubal dye test.

Hysteroscopy: An endoscopic procedure in which a doctor views the interior of the uterus.

Immunobead test: A test to detect the presence of anti-sperm antibodies.

Immunologic infertility: A condition in which the blood cells produce antibodies that attack sperm.

Impaired fecundity: Inability to sustain a pregnancy.

In-vitro fertilization (IVF): A technique in which eggs are harvested from the ovaries and mixed with sperm in a petri dish and allowed to fertilize to the pre-embryo stage (about 48 hours). At that point, pre-embryos are transferred to the uterus. IVF is also known as "test-tube" fertilization; sometimes used as a catchall term for GIFT, ZIFT, and other types of advanced reproductive technology.

Incompetent cervix: A condition in which the cervix opens prematurely under pressure from a growing fetus, resulting in a miscarriage.

Infertility: The inability to become pregnant (or make a woman pregnant) after one year of trying; or the inability to sustain a pregnancy naturally.

Infertility specialist: A medical doctor with advanced training in infertility or reproductive endocrinology; may or may not limit practice to infertility patients.

Intracervical insemination (ICI): A type of artificial insemination in which semen is injected into the cervix.

Intrauterine insemination (IUI): A type of AI in which washed semen is injected into the uterus.

Laparoscopy: A surgical procedure in which a rigid tube is inserted into the abdomen, usually through the navel, to allow the doctor to view or treat the reproductive organs.

Luteal phase defect: Insufficient progesterone secretion during the second half of the menstrual cycle.

Luteinizing hormone: A hormone produced by the pituitary to help stimulate the ovary to produce an egg follicle.

Miscarriage: Spontaneous pregnancy loss.

Motility: Term used to describe mobility, or swimming movements, of sperm.

Morphology: Term used to describe size and shape of sperm cells.

Mycoplasma: A type of bacterial infection that can cause infertility.

Oocyte: Medical term for egg.

Ovarian/follicle scan: An ultrasound scan of the ovaries used to track the growing egg sac or sacs.

Ovulation induction: Use of drugs to stimulate ovaries to grow one or more egg sacs in a given cycle.

Ovulatory dysfunction: Failure of the ovaries to produce naturally at least one egg per cycle; dysfunction can be temporary, intermittent, or ongoing.

Partial zona drilling (PZD): An experimental technique using microscopic instruments to drill a partial hole in the egg's shell to facilitate in-vitro fertilization.

Pelvic inflammatory disease (PID): An infection in the woman's reproductive system, usually caused by a sexually transmitted disease, which may damage the fallopian tubes and result in infertility; PID also may stem from a miscarriage, an abortion, childbirth, or an IUD.

Pituitary: Known as the "master gland," the pituitary is located in the base of the brain and is responsible for controlling other endocrine glands, which secrete a variety of hormones, including those involved in reproduction.

Polycystic ovarian disease (PCOD): A fertility-threatening disorder usually characterized by the growth of multiple cysts in the ovaries.

Caused by a hormonal imbalance, PCOD is also known as Stein-Leventhal syndrome. Symptoms include irregular periods, obesity, facial hair, and acne.

Post-coital test (PCT): Examination of cervical mucus for the presence of active sperm 8 to 24 hours after intercourse.

Pre-embryo: The stage of fertilization that occurs after two days; pre-embryos are transferred to the uterus in IVF.

Primary infertility: A condition in which a woman cannot become pregnant for the first time or carry her first baby to term because of a problem with her reproductive system or her partner's.

Progesterone: A female sex hormone secreted by the ovaries after ovulation; helps the process of implantation of a fertilized egg in the uterus.

Prolactin: A hormone secreted by the pituitary to stimulate the breasts to produce milk.

Prostaglandin: A type of fatty acid that behaves like a hormone; one of its functions is to stimulate uterine contractions during labor.

Reproductive endocrinologist: A medical doctor with advanced training in how hormones influence reproduction.

Retrograde ejaculation: An abnormality in which a man's semen flows backward into the bladder during orgasm.

Secondary infertility: A condition where a woman can naturally conceive and carry to term her first baby but is unable to get pregnant again or sustain a subsequent pregnancy.

Semen: Sperm-containing fluid produced in the testicles and ejaculated by the man during orgasm.

Semen analysis: A method of assessing the concentration, quality, and motility of sperm. Semen volume and other factors are measured before the microscopic examination.

Seminal vesicles: Glands in the testicles that produce fluids, which add volume to semen.

Sexual dysfunction: A man's inability to achieve or sustain an erection or to ejaculate during intercourse.

Sperm washing: Method of sperm preparation that eliminates dead sperm and debris from the seminal fluid.

Sperm-penetration test: A test in which human sperm is put in contact with cow cervical mucus or a hamster egg in a laboratory in order to estimate the sperm's penetration potential.

Sterility: Inability to become pregnant or to impregnate a woman, with or without medical intervention.

Superovulation: Production of many eggs, up to 15 or more, in a given cycle as a result of taking the ovulation-induction drug Pergonal. Inducing superovulation is common in IVF procedures and is sometimes used in AI.

Surrogate: A woman who carries someone else's baby to term; the baby may or may not be genetically related to the surrogate.

Test-tube baby: Colloquialism referring to babies born through IVF.

Testicular biopsy: Microscopic examination of a snippet of testicular tissue to determine, among other things, whether sperm are forming normally.

Testosterone: The primary male hormone responsible for sexual development as well as bone and muscle growth.

Tubal embryo (stage) transfer—TE(s)T: An ART procedure in which 48-hour-old pre-embryos are transferred to the fallopian tubes.

Uterine septum: A congenital abnormality in which tissue forms a wall dividing the uterine cavity in two.

Varicocele: A varicose vein, usually located just above the left testicle, that is believed to cause infertility in certain men by impairing sperm development.

Varicolectomy: A minor surgical procedure in which the varicocele is tied off through an incision in the lower abdomen; sperm improvement occurs in about 70 percent of cases.

Vas deferens: A small sperm duct leading from the testicles to the urethra.

Zygote intrafallopian transfer (ZIFT): An ART technique in which eggs fertilized to the zygote stage (after 24 hours—before the first cell division) in a petri dish are transferred to the fallopian tubes; sometimes called pronuclear stage transfer (PROST).

INDEX

ABOUT THE AUTHORS

SUSAN TREISER is currently co-director of IVF New Jersey in Somerset, New Jersey. She received her M.D. and Ph.D. from Georgetown University in Washington, D.C. She completed a residency in Obstetrics and Gynecology at UMDNJ–Robert Wood Johnson University Hospital as well as a fellowship in Reproductive Endocrinology and Infertility at Columbia-Presbyterian Hospital in New York. She currently lives in New Jersey with her husband and two sons, Matt and Adam.

ROBIN K. LEVINSON is a free-lance medical writer and editor with more than thirteen years in the newspaper field. The winner of some thirty national and state journalism awards, Ms. Levinson also teaches writing classes. She became pregnant after battling infertility for more than two years. She is currently researching a book on osteoporosis. She lives with her husband and daughter in New Jersey.